THE SIMPLE GUIDE
TO
SHEDDING THE POUNDS
AND
THE SIMPLE GUIDE
TO
PET ADOPTION

BY
WARREN BROWN

GOLDCOPY PUBLICATIONS
LONDON
2012

THE SIMPLE GUIDE
TO
SHEDDING THE POUNDS

AND

PET ADOPTION

BY

WARREN BROWN

ISBN 978-1-291-22708-6

Acknowledgments

To all those who assisted me with the research work
for this book.

DEDICATION

This book is dedicated to all those who believe that
they will be SLIM if they try.

INTRODUCTION

Dear Reader,

This book on the Secrets to shedding the Pounds will assist you on your way to a healthier and happier life.

Sincerely

Warren Brown
London
2012

This book on the Secrets to Shedding the Pounds will help you to...

1. Realize that you hold the key to a slimmer You.
2. You need to make changes in your lifestyle.
3. You need to control the types of food you eat.
4. You need to reduce your portions of food.
5. You need to build your self esteem.
6. You need will-power to make the changes in your life.
7. You need to be strict with your diet.
8. You need to keep time aside for regular exercises.
9. You need to eat more fruits and vegetables.
10. You need to discover the slimmer and more positive You.

How to Lose 10 Pounds in Three Days

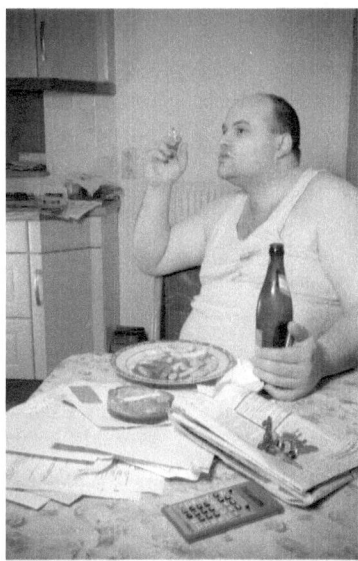

After all those nights of hard partying with your friends, you suddenly find yourself unable to fit on some of your clothes. Late night-outs can really take a toll on the body. What's worse is when you are expected to attend something important in a matter of days? This can really become a dilemma hard to get out of. Fret not because it is really possible to lose 10 pounds in three days.

Diet or Exercise

Of course the easiest answer to this is both. It is easier for those of you who've already established an exercise routine to shed off that extra weight fast. All you have to do is to follow your conventional routine while keeping in mind to follow a strict diet. Furthermore, altering the way you eat can be extremely helpful during those times when you really need to lose weight fast.

The key here is to compromise. If you are used to hard partying or eating whatever you want without taking a glance at the label, get ready to face the challenge of your life. Adapting to a healthy diet is very difficult but with determination you can definitely achieve a slimmer look.

Diet for Day 1

This type of diet consists of eating strictly these types of foods. This isn't a way of starving yourself but rather a method of improving your diet. Again, it is important not to vary from this diet otherwise you wouldn't achieve the desired results.

At breakfast during the first day, take one slice of toast and a half of grapefruit. You can partner these with two tablespoons of peanut butter as well as tea or coffee depending on your preference.

As for lunch, you can also drink coffee or tea coupled with half a cup of tuna and a slice of toast. Lastly, your dinner should consist of 3 ounces of any type of meat, a cup of beans and half a banana. You can also add one small apple and a cup of vanilla ice cream for dessert.

Diet for Day 2

For the second day's breakfast, partner your toast with boiled egg and half a banana. On the other hand, take a cup of cottage cheese, though you can substitute this with a slice of cheddar, another hard boiled egg and five pieces of saltine crackers for lunch.

Eat a cup of broccoli and ½ cup of carrots, half a banana and two pieces of hot dogs during dinner but remember not to include the buns. You can still consume one-half cup of vanilla ice cream for dessert.

Diet for Day 3

Your lunch meal for the second day should now be eaten for breakfast. This meal can be partnered with a piece of apple to help you through the day. As for your lunch, take a slice of toast and couple it with a piece of hard boiled egg.

Lastly for dinner, have a cup of tuna as well as half a piece of banana. You can also consume one-half to a cup of vanilla ice cream for dessert.

The most important aspect to remember while undergoing this type of diet is to never eat in between meals. If you feel hunger pangs, all you have to do is to drink a glass of cold water. In addition to this, remember to use only salt and pepper for seasoning and nothing else. This is guaranteed to help you lose ten pounds in three days. This is only intended to last for three days.

Once you achieve your desired results, be sure to continue to eat like you normally do.

Best Guidelines for a 10-Pound Weight Loss

Losing weight, as well all know, can bring tons of benefits most of which are long term. It can help improve the body's defenses against certain diseases as well as improve the psychological wellbeing. Wishing to shed a few extra pounds isn't that hard to realize. There are several guidelines for a 10-pound weight loss out there that you can surely utilize for your own advantage. Integrating these tips with your diet and exercise regimen can definitely help you lose weight for a shorter period of time.

Tell Others You Are On a Diet

Making your diet public is a form of affirmation. It is very hard to keep your diet a secret from others and there is not reason for you to do that. Telling others that you are on a diet can really help you in the long run. More people would be able to help you on your mission and you can depend on them more for morale support.

Motivation is the key to a successful diet. You can get this from those around you especially your from your friends and family. If you hear unsupportive comments, just brush them off and think of the positive effects of what you are doing.

Don't Forget to Drink Lots of Water

Water is obviously very helpful to the body. It can even be more helpful during diets. Water doesn't only help the body get rid of toxins and functions properly but also eliminate cravings. A sudden change in eating habits can cause unexpected cravings and hunger pangs. Water is very beneficial during these tough times.

A glass of cold water can effectively eliminate any of your cravings even for just a moment. Whenever you feel like eating but it is not time for your meal, grab a glass of water and drink until you feel the cravings melting away.

Purchase a Weighing Scale

You don't have to buy those large weighing beams that they use on the hospitals. There are several kinds of digital weighing scales available on your local hardware and electronic store. This is an important step in any diet; how else can you monitor your progress if you don't own a scale? Always remember to choose a brand that is known for its durability and accurateness.

You can either opt for a simple weighing scale that only has the basic ability to tell you how much you weight or something that has extra options like weight logging and comparison programs. The latter type of weighing scale is very helpful in telling you just how you are developing through the diet.

Make a Habit of Weighing Yourself Everyday

Once you bought a weighing scale, place it in your bedroom where you can easily access it after waking up. Most people only weight themselves once a week. Though this method is still effective, weighing yourself everyday can tell your daily progress. This is even more evident if you purchase a weighing scale that is accurate to the last detail. Always remember that a 180.8 is yesterday is different from 180.0. A weighing scale that can't tell your accurate weight even to the last decimal is less useful.

Losing as low as .8 in your weight is significant because it shows you exactly how your diet is working. Keep in mind that the diet is only as good as its results. Try to find more guidelines for a 10-pound weight loss or be creative and make one. You don't know how much they can help you achieve your goal.

Curb Your Hunger and Lose More Than 10 Pounds

The hardest part of changing the way you eat is to eliminate hunger pangs and cravings. The body has been so used to being full all the time that it causes you to eat in-between meals. This habit is certainly one of the leading causes of unnecessary weight gain. Most of the time, the food you eat during snacks are unhealthy although satiating. That is why it is important to know how to curb your hunger. Not only will this cause you to lose more weight and faster but also adapt a healthier lifestyle free of extra calories and fats.

Hunger, Satisfaction and Your Appetite

Most people believe that these three terms share a common meaning. That is not the case, however. The appetite doesn't necessarily mean hunger while hunger is not satiety or satisfaction. For starters, the appetite is more synonymous to cravings. It is characterized by a strong desire to eat a particular kind of food, i.e. "I have an appetite for chocolate cake right now."

On the other hand, hunger is a condition that usually occurs when the body is in dire need of nutrition. It is accentuated by shakiness, edginess, headache, and growling of the stomach. Lastly, satisfaction or satiety is simply the feeling of fulfillment or fullness. Most often, people stop eating when they are already satiated.

Healthy Eating

The three terms associated with eating (hunger, appetite and satisfaction) are affected by certain hormones of the body such as leptin, cholecystokin, ghrelin and insulin. All of these hormones cause the body to experience specific needs for nourishment. In addition, they affect a person's behavior and thoughts in relation to hunger, satisfaction and appetite.

One popular example of this is when a person feels an intense desire to eat more even if he or she already ate enough. During this circumstance, the endocrine gland produces excessive hormones that cause the person's satiety level. The overproduction of the hormone leptin can also induce intense appetite sometimes causing the person to desire highly unhealthy foods.

Managing Your Hunger

There are several ways that can help you manage your hunger effectively. Creating irregular eating periods can cause the body to adapt to the new meal schedule. This doesn't mean, though, that you should eat erratically but rather scatter meals all throughout the day.

Consuming less starchy and sugar-filled meals can also decrease your hunger levels. Excessive consumption of sugar can cause fluctuations of your blood sugar that will not only affect the way you lose weight but also cause eventual diabetes. Lastly, simple elimination of hunger and appetite stimuli can help manage the weight better. Make sure you decrease the amount of unhealthy desserts and snacks at your home.

Managing Your Satiety

It is important to know that there are several factors that contribute to increase satiety. One is lessening the time gap between meals or eating every two to three hours. Also, eating a high protein diet can also cause effective satiety since protein has been known to cause satiety.

Fiber, which helps digestion and clean the digestive tract, can also cause prolonged satiety since the body needs more time to digest fiber enriched foods. Incorporating fiber and protein rich food in your diet can effectively curb your hunger.

Diet Makeover Tips to Help You Lose 10 Pounds or More

It is certainly difficult to look for a diet plan that suits your lifestyle. However, you must remember that going on a diet is a lifestyle change itself. You must be willing to make early sacrifices in order to get you nearer to your goal. Luckily, there are several diet makeover tips you can use to help ease the transition. These are by no means diet routines but rather a way of changing your eating habit healthily and gradually.

With the number of diet techniques sprouting here and there, you definitely need a helping hand in choosing the right one. These tips can help you land the perfect regimen for you as well as shorten the time it will take you to lose those extra pounds.

Plan Your Meals

The first and most important part of transitioning into a healthy lifestyle is planning correctly what you must eat. This is can be daunting task especially for those who are always on the go. You must remember, though, that this step is important in helping you get used to the new eating habits.

Everyday, you must remember to plan you meal before you even take them. For instance, before eating breakfast, you must set up a desired meal plan the night before. Pack your food beforehand to ensure that you get the right measurements required by whatever diet method you are taking. The same goes for your lunch and dinner. As you continue with the diet, you wouldn't believe how easy and beneficial it is to plan a meal beforehand.

Purge Your Fridge and Pantry

This is probably one of the hardest sacrifices you have to make in order to lose weight. It is time for you to open your fridge and other food storage and purge them of any unhealthy food. Throw that ice cream, cake, chips, candies and everything that are unhealthy, and replace them with healthier alternatives, like whole wheat pretzels and crackers, breads and pastas.

Purchase Guilt-Free Snacks

The on-going need to stay fit and healthy brought about the creation of guilt-free snacks that you can munch on without worrying of gaining extra pounds. This is extremely helpful if you still are having a hard time giving up your in-between meal sessions or fighting those nasty cravings.

Some of these healthier alternatives include almonds, dried fruits, sugar-free desserts and more. Even your favourite condiments now have their organic counterparts, which are free of the chemicals sometimes attributed to weight gain.

Drinks and beverages that pack a lot of calories should also be lessened, if not eliminated. Instead of drinking carbonated sodas and commercially packed fruit juices, opt for healthier diet sodas and freshly squeezed juices. Also remember to add a sugar-free packet to your bottled water whenever you drink one.

Choose White Meat Instead of Red

The best way to lose weight without eliminating protein is to choose white meat over red. Skinless chicken breasts are very lean and contain high quality protein, which is essential in losing weight. Baking them can further enhance their nutritional value.

Another one of the diet makeover tips you can use is to substitute fish meat for your pork or beef. Fish meat is healthier and contains high quality fatty acids that can help improve heart and other bodily functions. Nevertheless, remember to include protein in your diet to create balance.

Four Reasons Why It Is Hard to Lose 10 Pounds

Losing the slightest amount of weight is tough. Losing ten pounds is even tougher. If you are not careful enough, the lost weight will come back to haunt you. Remember that gaining weight is a lot easier than losing weight for almost everybody. Aside from those who are blessed with good genes allowing them not to gain any weight no matter how plenty they eat, us mere mortals will find it hard to lose even a single pound without the much needed effort. That is why knowing the reasons why it is hard to lose 10 pounds or less is important.

Getting behind that reasons of your weight loss struggle is the key in eliminating some of the effort needed to lose weight. At the same time, some of these causes can also be the reason why some people gain weight faster than anyone else. It is time to explore the factors that play a major role in managing weight.

Physical Problems

Many people don't realize that they can easily gain weight due to some underlying conditions. There are plenty of medical conditions that can contribute to weight gain. Some of these include pituitary disorders, blood sugar imbalance, and a relatively low thyroid hormone.

Malfunctions in the adrenal gland can also cause some people to gain weight faster. Liver and kidney disease can also become a factor. Even drugs that are used to cure such diseases can also cause some people to gain weight especially if the drugs have a fluid retention side-effect. That is why it is important to go to a doctor first before even deciding to lose weight in order to properly assess the right course of action.

High Levels of Stress

The popular Yo-Yo dieting, which has been a trend to most celebrities nowadays, is mostly caused by huge level of stress. Stress can affect the weight of a person; either losing or gaining weight can be caused by stress. The body can also cause stress by producing stress hormones, like epinephrine and cortisol in huge amounts.

These two hormones can cause the abdomen to store more fats than usual. Avoiding the production of these stress-inducing hormones must be dealt with externally through avoiding stressors whether from work or at home. Finding relaxing activities can also help the body eliminate stress.

Body's Toxicity Levels

If the body absorbs too much toxins, it will need those extra pounds to dilute them. This is why it is important to opt for organic foods. Not only are they healthier but contains fewer toxins from chemicals. Conventional methods of farming require chemicals to fight against pests attracted to produce. Spraying pesticides is a normal ritual when growing crops. However, this practice causes health problem, which eventuates to weight gain or inability to lose weight.

Addictions to Food and Beverage

Let's face it, all of us love food. However, the excessive love for food and beverage obviously causes weight gain and obesity. Furthermore, addiction to drugs especially narcotics can cause the imbalances to your weight. Some chemicals like those from marijuana can cause the body to crave for more food than usual.

Alcohol addiction can also cause weight gain due to the alcohol's ability to dehydrate the body. This would result to an increase need to eat and drink. Aside from those, excessive use of sugar on food and drinks can cause the body to gain weight faster. Depending on such unhealthy habits is one of the major reasons why it is hard to lose 10 pounds or even less.

Easy Techniques to Lose 10 Pounds in One Week

Losing extra pounds gradually is the healthiest way to keep in shape. Instead of wanting to shave off those extra pounds in a day or two, which can be a very daunting endeavour, a pound or two each day is a healthier alternative. There are several ways to lose 10 pounds in one week but only a handful of them work. More so, some of those diets even subtly suggest going to extremes like not eating anything at all.

If you are unsure of what kind of diet regimen you should undertake to help you lose weight, here is a one-week meal plan you can try. Just follow these few simple steps and see yourself slimmer in a span of one week.

Day One

On the first day of the diet, it is important to condition the body. You can do this by taking a detox diet. Not only will this help the body lose weight faster but cleanse it as well. Start the day by mixing a cup of lemon juice, slices of ginger and honey with one cup of water.

It is helpful to prepare a mixture of this detox drink that can last the whole day. This way whenever you are hungry, all you have to do is to drink a cup of the detox mixture.

Day Two

It is important to limit the amount of food you eat to help your body lose weight fast. However, don't forget to eat healthy and incorporate lots of fruits and vegetables to your meals. You can also eat meat but remember to chose lean ones or opt for white meat like chicken or fish instead.

Day Three

Once you got used to your new diet, start adding two pieces of apples and a cup of black beans to your meals. You can also substitute the beans for the meats. This can jumpstart your fibre intake, which in turn helps for healthy weight loss.

Day Four

During the fourth day of the diet, start eating heavy breakfast mostly consisting of grains and cereals. Again, fibre is very important because it really does wonders for the digestive system. As for your dinner, remember to eat the meal before seven o'clock. Eating after seven in the evening or hours before sleep can restrict the body from properly digesting your meal.

Day Five

It is important to realize just how much calorie you consume during the previous three days especially now that you have established a healthy diet. Once you are aware of this, try to scatter your meals all throughout the day. Eating five to six small meals is a great way to help you lose weight.

Day Six

During this time, you must be able to limit your sugar and fat intake. If not, try to limit your consumption further. There are other healthier alternatives for these kinds of foods. For instance, instead of eating ice cream for dessert, eat yogurt. They are healthier and provide the body with helpful and healthy bacteria.

Day Seven

Eat fresh fruits instead of packaged juices. Another healthier alternative is to drink freshly squeezed juices without additives and flavourings. You can even stop drinking juice altogether and rather opt for a healthier green tea.

This kind of diet can be prolonged if you want to continuously lose weight. Once you lose 10 pounds in one week, remember that maintaining this type of healthy diet can prevent you from gaining weight.

Helpful Methods to Help You Lose Those Extra 10 Pounds

A dieter should grab hold of any helpful advice he or she can gain access to. Although most of the tips on dieting is a dime a dozen, there are a chosen few that can really provide significant results. As a person on a weight loss mission, you should consider applying any methods to help you lose those extra 10 pounds easily on your daily diet routine.

Use a Mirror When Eating

This doesn't mean that you should hold a mirror while you are munching your dinner. You should place a mirror in front of your dining table or anywhere you can see yourself easily whenever you eat. Some studies reveal that people who constantly see themselves in the mirror slash their food consumption to as much as one-third of their usual eating habits.

Seeing yourself in the mirror can have a significant reaction to the brain which has been set for a specific goal. This would help remind yourself the reason why you are trying to lose weight in the first place.

Put More Vegetables on Your Plate

Seeing a full plate can definitely help you enjoy the meal more. However, filling your plate with unhealthy foods is not the right way to lose weight. Instead of putting too much meat on your dinner plate, increase your meal by replacing them with vegetables. Choosing vegetables that can take more space of the plate, like cauliflower, broccoli, tomatoes and carrots, is definitely helpful in creating a full plate.

Eat Water-Rich Vegetables

There are studies showing that eating more vegetables that are rich in water can help reduce your daily calorie consumption. Such vegetables that you should think about eating everyday are cucumbers, zucchini, tomatoes and more. You can also opt for salads and soups instead of eating solid foods to help your body lose weight faster. Although these foods don't have the same advantage as water, they can still do the trick in keeping your stomach full for a longer period.

Colour Instead of White

It has been found that white foods have the tendency to cause the body to gain more weight. Although it is unhealthy not to eat carbohydrates, lessening your daily consumption is advisable. Also, try not to consume food that are rich in white sugar and flour, which can definitely ruin your blood sugar levels thus causing weight gain instead of weight loss.

If you are fond of eating rice, choose the brown variant, which is healthier than the white one. Whole wheat breads and cereals are also very helpful in fending off weight gain and promoting healthy weight loss.

Eat Most of Your Meals At Home

This is the time for you to prepare and eat your food at home. You must remember not to eat outside regularly. Eating your food at the comfort of your own home can help you thoroughly monitor the food you consume. You just don't know what they put on those restaurant foods.

Take Time Chewing Your Food

Eating hastily can cause bloating and gas – this is a common truth. On the contrary, eating slowly promotes healthy digestion. Don't depend on your stomach to do all the hard work. Chew your food slowly. Taking some time to chew is definitely helpful in proper nutrient absorption. Furthermore, this allows your brain to tell you accurately that you are full and no longer need food.

This is one of the most useful methods to help you lose those extra 10 pounds in a matter of weeks.

How Diet Supplements Can Help You Lose 10 Pounds

A person undergoing a major weight loss program sometimes lack the daily recommended vitamins and minerals. This is because some diet plans require dieters to limit their food intake thus causing a slightly significant decrease in vitamin and mineral consumption. Luckily, there are supplements that can fill in the gap. It is a common fact that diet supplements can help you lose 10 pounds or even more. These pills are one of the most important parts of any diet plans.

However, you must first know the facts of these supplements before you go on taking some of them. Diet supplements are, fortunately, rarely detrimental to the health.

They're there to Help You

Anyone can benefit from dietary supplements. No matter what your goals are, be it weight loss or overall health and wellness, these pills can help you in your journey. The supplements can even help you even if the diet you choose is sub par from the other widely popular ones.

You must remember, though, the golden rule in taking such supplements: "No dietary pill can help you solve all your problems; they are magic pills." They are called supplements for exactly that reason only – to supplement any deficiency in your diet. There are supplements for virtually any kind of help you need: from anti-aging and skin health to weight loss and muscle toning.

Facts Regarding DietarySupplements

Anyone who has been using dietary supplements for a very long time knows that these pills are not FDA-approved since they are neither considered food nor drugs. Thus, you must realize that the labels on any supplements you see do not guarantee accurate results or even contents. For instance, a 100mg vitamin C tablet may contain less than 100mg.

This is why it is important to choose the label that you trust or have been trusted by several people for many years. Don't be cheap when it comes to supplements because the supplement is only as good as the manufacturer.

Supplements for Overall Health

Those who are satisfied with how they look or what they weigh concentrate on maintaining and better managing their health. Some of the most common supplements for this type of goal are vitamin and mineral supplements. A multivitamin supplements that contains every vitamin you need everyday can provide the essential micronutrients. Furthermore, these types of pills can even promote healthy metabolic rates.

The antioxidant supplements are also another type of dietary supplement. They are taken to help the body fight free radicals that are everywhere. Those who actively participate in rigorous aerobic exercises can definitely benefit from these supplements.

Weight Loss Supplements

Partnering your diet and exercise regimen can help achieve desired results. These types of supplements are easily the number one dietary pills out there due to the increase need to be healthy. It is very healthy to consider taking a weight loss supplement to jumpstart your weight loss program. Doing so would also be helpful if you have set a specific time frame for your diet and exercise.

Diet supplements can help you lose 10 pounds or more if you take them regularly or within the duration of your diet. One popular kind of these supplements is the green-tea diet supplement which provides not only antioxidants but fat-burning agents as well.

Why You Can't Shed 10 Pounds in Two Days

Wanting to shed 10 pounds in two days is probably the extreme desire one could have with regards to weight loss. Though you can still lose a relatively good amount of weight in the span of two days, the toll this can put to the body can be disastrous. Yet most people still seek to lose 10 pounds or more the shortest duration.

On the brighter side of things, a two-day diet is still doable. Although the diet techniques aimed at this sort of rapid weight loss can be difficult to do, with willingness and determination nothing is impossible.

The Cyclone Diet

One popular kind of diet that promises to deliver results in just two short days is the Cyclone Diet. This quick-fix diet can still help you lose weight but it is more likely to improve the body's detox methods. In short, a cyclone diet is more of a detox diet.

The diet mainly includes a pack of powder that, when mixed with water, must be consumed three time in the course of 48 hours. The Cyclone Diet is commercially available and even contains helpful herbs to prevent you from fainting if you decide to fast during the diet.

Eating and Exercising

During the course of the Cyclone Diet, you can still eat – fasting is only optional. However, bear in mind that there is a limitation to what you can actually consume during the two days of the diet. For starters, you are not allowed to eat meat but instead only raw or steamed vegetables. No caffeine should also be observed during the diet as well as sugar free deserts mainly consisting of yogurt. Salt must also be minimized and prevented if necessary.

Aside from eating the right food, you must also combine it with a two day period of mild exercise routines. For the first day of the diet, you are advised to do a five-mile bicycle ride as well as two miles of running. On the next day, fourteen miles of bicycling is required combined with a light dumbbell routine for about thirty minutes. You must also remember to combine the two-day exercise routine with some mild abdominal crunches.

Side Effects of the Diet

Even though the Cyclone Diet can be considered extreme, the side effects range from mild to none depending if you proceeded with fasting or not. The only obvious effect of the diet is regular bowel movement all throughout the day. For this reason, you must clear your entire schedule and dedicate yourself to the diet. You'll most likely make several trips to the bathroom.

Possible Results of the Diet

The side effects only prove that the Cyclone Diet is 90% cleansing and 10% weight loss. Remember that the weight loss benefit is only secondary to the detoxification. Fortunately, cleansing has its own benefits to the body. It obviously cleans the body of toxins and excess fat deposits as well as condition the diet for further weight loss regimen.

Just don't expect to shed 10 pounds in two days because the most you can lose is two to four pounds. This is still fairly substantial compared to a 10-pound weight loss in two weeks. However before making the diet a regular habit, you must know that the Cyclone Diet is not designed for prolonged usage.

How to Lose 10 Pounds If You Are Over 40

People, especially women, nearing their prime must realize that losing weight is the same no matter what the age may be. For those wondering if it is possible to lose 10 pounds if you are over 40, yes it is. The dietary and exercise routines remain the same. The fundamentals are not altered – even the goals remain true. There is certainly a diversity of methods you can take in order to lose weight effectively.

Use a Pedometer

One way to exercise is to climb a set of steps. Experts agree that a daily 3000-step exercise routine is helpful in burning fats. Fortunately, a pedometer can help you with such task. A pedometer is simply an electronic device that can help you count the steps you take. The electronic device does this by detecting the motion of the hips. However, before buying one you must first know how to pick the right device that can provide you with accuracy.

Firstly, you should not be cheap. Several market outlets offer cheap or free pedometer – these devices can't provide you with proper readings. Next, you should learn how to program that device and concentrate mainly on counting the steps you take.

Add Imaginary Calories

In case you set a daily calorie intake you can follow, it is always helpful to add an imaginary 10 calorie to everything you are about to eat. For instance, if you have set your daily calorie intake to 1,600, you should be able to know just how much calorie each food you eat has. If the label says 130 calories per serving, add 10 or 15 imaginary calorie to that to make it 140-145. This can ultimately help you achieve your daily calorie intake since chances are, your estimation is accurate.

Spread Your Meals

During normal circumstances, there are only three basic mealtimes: breakfast, lunch and dinner. If you want to effectively shed off extra pounds, add three to four meals in between. However, make these meals smaller than normal. Divide your breakfast to two as well as your lunch and dinner. Eating small can help you avoid hunger pangs in between meals, which is the most common reason of weight loss failure.

Take Time to Walk

If you allow yourself to do some simple cardio routines everyday, you would surely slowly lose weight. The easiest cardio exercise, and not to mention cheapest, is to walk. Many people find it beneficial to take some time everyday for a leisurely walk. A thirty to forty-five-minute walk can help you burn as much as 600 calories everyday.

Buy a Pair of Pants Three Sizes Smaller

Having a goal is helpful in losing weight. Why not materialize this goal in the form of a pair of pants? Buying a pair of expensive pants two to three sizes smaller than the ones you wear can provide you inspiration. This can motivate you to reach your goal. Make sure that you buy the most expensive you can find to make you regret not being able to wear them in case you fail your weight loss program.

There are more ways to lose 10 pounds if you are over 40. All you need to have is patience and determination. Once you achieve your goal, be sure to remove all the clothes that remind you of your previous weight from your closet. Purchase a new set of wardrobe to encourage you to maintain your new figure.

Exercises to Help You Reduce 10 Pounds

The stomach is one of the most problematic areas to deal with when trying to lose weight. Fortunately, there are several exercises that target that area. Exercises to help you reduce 10 pounds are certainly effective in helping you achieve the figure you want. You can definitely reap the benefits of exercising regularly if you are truly persistent and committed.

Climbing Steps

One of the most effective ways to not only reduce stomach fat but also improve quads and other leg muscles is climbing. You don't have to engage in tedious hiking trips in order to do this. If you have a set of steps in your house, you can repeatedly climb it for at least thirty minutes.

Another effective way to do this is to use a treadmill. Treadmills can be inclined to increase the intensity of the workout. All you have to do is to incline the platform for at least ten to fifteen degrees and exercise for about fifteen minutes. You can gradually increase the time you spend on the exercise as you progress.

Squatting

Squats are other excellent exercise routines to help burn fats on the stomach. These types of exercises can help reduce your waist size by effectively burning huge amounts of calories. Take note that squats can create a huge oxygen deficit in order to improve the body's method of burning fat.

To start the exercise, first choose a part of your house where you cannot be disturbed or at least bump on any furniture. Start by squatting up and down while making sure that the tips of your fingers are able to touch the ground. This is different from other types of squatting wherein you place your hands behind your head. The exercise can be very effective if you do at most 100 repetitions in less than five minutes.

You can increase the intensity of the exercise by doing 200 repetitions in less than ten minutes. Just make sure that you progress gradually and not hastily to allow the body time to adjust.

The Vacuum Exercise

This is a fairly easy but effective way to reduce stomach fat. You don't have to have any fancy equipment for this since all you need to do is to maintain a pose for a few seconds. You can start by sucking in your belly button until you feel it seemingly touching your spine. It doesn't necessarily have to be that intense though if you can't handle it. As long as you can prolong the pose for 50 to 60 seconds, you are doing it correctly.

After holding it for the required amount of time, rest and then repeat. Do this everyday for at least 20 minutes. This exercise is guaranteed to trim at least an inch of your waist in less than a month. Some even lose as much as three inches.

Bicycle Crunches

Bicycle crunches is one of the most effective exercises to help you reduce 10 pounds and trim off that excess fat on your stomach. Start by lying on a comfortable mat and placing your hands behind your head. Slowly touch the tip of your right elbow with your left knee. Do the same for your left elbow and right knee. Gradually increase the speed of the exercise all the while tensing your abdomen. You can effectively burn significant amounts of calories everyday by performing the exercise for at least fifteen minutes.

How to Lose 10 Pounds or More Permanently

After months of struggling to lose weight, it can be a pain when suddenly you gain them back. Make sure that you don't waste the effort you placed on losing weight by going back to your old eating habits. Losing weight should be a long time commitment right from the beginning. Fortunately, there are several ways for you to lose 10 pounds or more permanently without the fear of gaining them ever again.

Choose a Cookie-Cutter Diet

Choosing cookie-cutter diets is the best way to go. Never fall for diet regimes that offer extra gimmicks. People who tend to follow these kinds of diet cannot completely commit thus causing failure. When you are aiming for weight loss, look for a no-nonsense diet that can guide you through everyday and provide healthy tips and techniques.

Also, make sure that you choose an inexpensive diet plan or one that can be maintained through a small amount of money. Diets tend to be more expensive when they become hyped up and more popular. Since many people are using the diet, the creators therefore have the reason to increase the price for more profit. This often results in gaining the lost weight again upon failure to adhere to the expensive diet.

Choose a Well-Balanced Diet

The basic aspect of a diet is balance. You can also measure the success rate of a diet plan if you notice how it effectively balances the kinds of food you must. It is important to realize that a diet should equally favor all healthy foods and not promote one kind from the other. This is why a diet that concentrates on a specific type of food, like high-protein or all fibre diet, rarely succeed – not to mention it is unhealthy.

Lessening your daily calorie intake doesn't mean you have to favour one requirement from the other. There should be an equal distribution of fats, protein and carbohydrates in the food you eat everyday in order to successfully and healthily lose weight.

Have the Right Attitude

Your attitude plays an important role not only in the success of the diet but also the maintenance of the newly acquired weight. Once you have managed to slash a significant number from your weight, you should always remember to motivate yourself to maintain it or even lose more. Always tell yourself that you can prolong this kind of lifestyle. If you can't, just think of the health benefits that you have achieved and you can achieve in the future.

Having the right attitude also means moderation. You don't have to be a hardcore dieter for the rest of your life. Even though dieting requires some sort of self-control and control towards the food you eat, you do not have to be meticulous up to the last detail. For the first time since the diet, you can relax and this is the right time for you to do so. Maintain the weight and think of losing later. You'll be doing your body a favour by lessening the stress sometimes brought about by extreme dietary routines.

Always Be Consistent

In any kind of diet, whether weight loss or maintenance, consistency is very important. Without the proper mindset, success cannot be realized. Consistency is very beneficial to the body. When you managed to cut calories from your daily consumption, the body becomes used to the change. By being consistent with this calorie decrease, you are allowing the body to adapt even further.

This type of consistency in the diet will cause you to lose 10 pounds or more permanently.

How to Lose 10 Pounds the Fast and Easy Way

Most people are naturally impatient. As humans, we have the innate desire to have anything we want in an instant; by hook or by crook, so to speak. This is especially true when it comes to weight loss. With the constant pressure of losing and maintaining weight, most of us resort to unhealthy measures. However, you don't need to reach new heights just to lose 10 pounds the fast and easy way.

Health and fitness is a multi-billion dollar industry. Almost everyday new weight loss products are advertised on the television; new and sometimes even seemingly absurd techniques to help lose weight is created. Unfortunately, many people bite into this kind of propaganda. Lest we forget the rudiments of staying fit and healthy, these faux techniques will continue their placebo effects.

The Importance of Exercising

Experts cannot stress enough the importance of exercise. Mere dieting can be effective but it is extremely unhealthy. Losing weight without exercising can cause adverse effects to the body. This is for the reason that the body will not be able to adjust properly to the newly adapted eating habits. The skin, for instance, must be flexible enough for weight loss so as not to produce any marks and sag.

Probably the quintessential question when it comes to exercising is "how much time should you devote for exercise?" Basically, as low as thirty minutes of exercise each day is necessary. This can help you get used to the new change in your daily routine. Since losing weight requires a certain amount of dedication, doing it gradually and in progression is very helpful.

The Types of Important Exercises

There are two kinds of exercises that you should take part in: cardio and strength exercises. These two are important in their own ways. Cardio exercises can help you endure strength training exercises longer. It helps you manage your breathing methods better and improves your overall cardiovascular system.

Coupling cardio training with strength exercises is also very helpful. Building lean muscles is helpful in burning calories. This is for the mere fact that muscles require more calories to maintain as compared to fats. No calorie is wasted when you have leaner muscles.

Dieting and Eating Healthy

The common diet faux pas is starvation. When you are trying to lose weight, it doesn't necessarily require you to starve yourself. You don't have to lessen your meals but rather improve them by incorporating healthy food. Dieting is all about eating right and staying within the bounds of what is considered healthy. You don't want to lose weight while putting your body at risk.

Eating foods that are high in fiber and essential vitamins and minerals are extremely crucial.

Substitute your plain rice to brown rice for a healthier alternative and cake desserts to fruits and fresh juices.

Managing Your Hunger Pangs

For someone who is new to dieting, exercising and overall losing weight, managing hunger pangs can be a pain. Cravings are very hard to address since they require more than determination to completely eliminate them. What you can do is to buy healthier snacks, which you can eat whenever you feel hungry in between meals.

Soon enough you would be able to completely eliminate your cravings. Not only will you be able to lose 10 pounds the fast and easy way by doing so but also maintain and manage your weight more effectively.

Lose 10 Pounds by Knowing These Diet Myths

Many people follow a diet for wrong reasons. They are so caught up with the hype that they forget to inspect everything that the diet claims. There are several diet myths out there that you should know. Realizing these diet myths can help you in a successful weight loss journey. Don't let yourself be tricked again by the hooplas most diets cause to achieve popularity.

Eating Carbohydrates is Not That Bad

Many diets claim that if you don't eat carbohydrates you will lose more weight. Wrong. You still need carbohydrates to help you survive the day. This type of myth is commonly found in those no-carb or low-carb diets. The popular Atkins diet even carries this type of myth too.

The topic of 'energy consumed versus energy burned' is an on-going debate. Carbohydrates, in excess, can surely be attributed for weight gain though this doesn't mean that you should eliminate them at all from your diet. A wonderful balance of protein, fat and carbohydrate is the key to a healthy and successful weight loss.

Exercising is only for the Overweight

People usually take exercise for granted. Those who are not considered overweight or obese often neglect exercising at all. This should not be the case because exercising is important not only in losing weight but maintaining it as well. Even if you don't look overweight, you can still have more fat than those who share your body type. It is important to consider the fat to muscle mass ratio.

Exercise regularly if you don't want to develop serious medical conditions. Even as low as a thirty-minute jog everyday can help maintain and manage your weight properly. Remember that the main cause of heart problems is fat build up and you can definitely eliminate this through effective exercise routines.

Eating Habits Is Not Related to Exercise

Considering exercise and eating habit as two separate things is the common mistake most people make. Even if you exercise regularly, you must still watch what you eat. Your eating habits and exercise must go hand-in-hand. What use is your exercise if you eat unhealthily? You'll just wear yourself out from exercising everyday and gaining back the weight also everyday. Being mindful of what you eat can help make your rigorous exercise routines more effective.

You Must Exercise Hard to Beat off Weight Gain

There are many kinds of diet regimen that require you to regularly push yourself to the limits in terms of exercising even if you managed to achieve your weight goal. They advice you to continuously workout harder in order to avoid gaining back the lost weight. You don't have to follow this myth.

Once you have managed to achieve your desired weight and want to maintain it, you can lessen your workout routine. Instead of going to the gym everyday for three-hours, you can lessen it to an hour three times a week. This would definitely clear up some time for you to do more important things you need to attend to.

What you can also do is to choose a lighter cardio routine, like one-hour brisk walking or thirty-minute treadmill exercise, over a more intense aerobic exercise. You can definitely lose weight in a matter of weeks if you choose not to follow several diet myths out there.

Lose 10 Pounds with These Diet Techniques You Can Do Everyday

Casual dieters are those who aren't that concerned with how much they weigh but rather settle on maintaining a healthy lifestyle. There are several ways to manage health but it is even more helpful to use these techniques to lose those unwanted pounds. Whether you are a casual dieter or someone with a mission, applying diet techniques you can do everyday can help you achieve a slimmer figure.

It is important to go on a diet that isn't much of a hindrance to your daily activities. It is very helpful indeed to adapt healthier eating habits without the need to sacrifice important activities you need to attend to daily.

Be Active

Most people eat too much due to extreme ennui and stress. The latter can even cause unnecessary and potentially unhealthy eating habits that you must avoid. It is very crucial to find an activity that you enjoy to battle boredom and stress. In addition, don't choose activities, which cannot do anything for your diet. For instance, instead of watching television whenever you are doing nothing, why not go on a leisurely walk?

Activities that can improve your weight loss program are truly helpful in battling the stress that comes with it. The next time you feel bored during weekends, take your family and go swimming or invite your friends for a friendly match of bowling.

Always Be Optimistic

The main enemy of a successful weight loss routine is negative thinking. Just because you fail to lose weight last week doesn't mean you have to give up altogether. On the contrary, you must strive harder to lose more weight. The mistakes you might have made during the previous week should teach you how to improve and develop as a dieter. This would further propel you near your diet goals.

Self-affirmation is also important during diets. This helps you create a positive mindset and motivates you to success in losing weight. Everyday you wake up, don't forget to tell yourself that you can lose weight and you will succeed.

Go Mediterranean

A Mediterranean diet has been known to provide a lot of helpful benefits because the cuisine incorporates a lot of healthy dishes sans the butter and margarine. Make it a point in your eating habits to include any Mediterranean dish you can cook. There are several easy-to-do dishes that provide tons of health and weight loss benefits.

In addition, instead of using fat-filled condiments opt for spicy flavorings. Spicy flavorings are known to possess satiating qualities. In fact, some of them, especially hot chili, contain vitamins and minerals that promote weight loss as well as boost the immune system. Next time you dine out, choose restaurants that are known for their Mediterranean dishes or simply opt for salsa instead of mayonnaise for your dish.

Limit Your Time Eating With Friends

This can be tough and quite contradictory to some diet tips saying that you need people around you for a successful weight. In reality, you still need those people for morale support just don't take them with you at the table. Recent studies show that we are likely to eat more than usual when we are in the presence of a group or eating out within a group.

This is simply because we tend to spend more time at the table when we are in a group. To fight this, use the time you spend after chewing for talking. This can definitely cut down the food you eat and make you eat slower. This is one of the diet techniques you can do everyday that saves you tons of calories.

Lose More Than 10 Pounds in 10 Days

There is nothing like the prospect of losing more than 10 pounds in 10 days. However, most people seem to lack the motivation they need to start a weight loss regimen. To jumpstart your diet, you would be glad to know that a juice fasting diet can help you achieve a healthier figure.

Benefits of the Juice Fasting Diet

A typical juice fasting diet provides several long-term benefits. Some of these advantages include: an improvement in the body's ability to detoxify and expel harmful toxins, increase the metabolic rate and develop the body's ability to absorb nutrition properly. More so, this kind of diet can eventually eliminate addictions and cravings.

Planning Your Diet

It is important to start on a weekend because the first two days of the diet is the hardest. This would give you a lot of time to deal possible food withdrawal symptoms and feel the purging effects of the diet. Additionally, make sure you stock a number of distractions in your house. Movies, books and games are excellent distractions.

If you are employed, plan the diet on a week that is particularly less stressful. For instance, pick a week when you are most likely to handle less assignments and projects. The diet can be stressful on its own. You don't want to put more stress on the body as this can hinder your success rate.

Mixing the Juice for the Diet

This is the most important part of the diet. Firstly, make sure you are equipped with an excellent juicer since this would be your friend for the duration of the diet. Make sure it can handle juicing in frequencies of six to eight times a day.

As for the type of juice, there are plenty you could choose from. For starters, you can opt for the Lemonade Diet or the Master Cleanse, which consists of maple syrup, lemonade with a spike of cayenne pepper. A basic 2:2:.5 ratio of the mixture should be mixed with double ounces of water is enough for one glass.

Make sure you drink the mixture each time you feel hungry. Don't be afraid of depriving yourself of food because the nutritional content of the juice is enough to supply you with a daily dose of vitamins and minerals. Plus, it is actually very satisfying. It is important not to deviate from the diet otherwise you'll fail.

Sailing through the Diet

The most important attitude you should posses during the diet is patience. The juice fasting diet will definitely test you during the first week. To survive this, always be optimistic and believe that you are doing something good to your body.

In addition, make sure you drink plenty of water during the course of the diet instead of relying on the juice to keep you hydrated. It is very important to drink lots of water to your body detoxify even more effectively. If you follow this routine, you are sure to lose more than 10 pounds in 10 days. After achieving the desired results, remember to go back to your regular eating habits.

Just make sure that you eat healthy and add a daily exercise routine to maintain your weight, lose more weight and prevent your body from gaining back the lost weight.

Methods to Help You Shed Extra 10 Pounds in Two Weeks

Weight loss especially if you are overweight can be extremely hard to achieve. There are the uncontrollable cravings and the lack of determination to achieve a weight goal. These and more factors play important roles in successful weight loss. What makes weight loss harder is setting unrealistic goals. If you desire to lose pounds in a matter of days, you should be prepared to handle the pressure. Sometimes to shed extra 10 pounds in two weeks or even every one and a half weeks is a healthier and easier choice.

This is very true to those who find it extremely hard to lose weight. Obesity is a major problem of our society and it is a never-ending battle to those who suffer from it. That is why moderation and proper adaptation to a diet and exercise regimen is important.

Aerobics and Cardio Exercises

Losing weight involves several kinds of exercise regimens. So much so that intensive aerobics exercise and other kinds of cardio training are important. Deciding to lose weight requires determination and especially dedication. Enrolling in a gym program that offers aerobics classes should be the first step in your weight loss program.

On the other hand, it is sometimes hard to dedicate yourself in such a program. What you can do is to try working out on your own. Simply by walking everyday for three hours can help you lose weight. Then, gradually increase the intensity of your cardio workout by changing it to running or even swimming.

Strength Training Programs

Aside from aerobics exercises, strength training is also important. Be sure to couple your daily cardio training with intensive strength training. These kinds of exercises require you to build lean muscles, which is helpful in burning calories. Weight lifting as well as stretching and crunches can easily help you build the type of body you want.

Detox Dieting

Detox dieting is a diet that is not only helpful in managing your weight but in cleansing your body as well. Detox dieting is continuously becoming popular due to its effectiveness. Detoxifying your body is very easy. This type of diet only requires you to always drink a mixture of lemon juice, honey, ginger and water everyday.

However, detox dieting should only be done during the first few days of your weight loss journey. It is not in any way should be maintained or even prolonged. This is because detox dieting is only used to help your body clean and condition itself for the coming intense weight management.

Eating Healthy

Combining exercise with a healthy diet is an age old truth in the issue of weight loss. Time and time again, experts always suggest everyone to eat healthy. Just how can you consider your eating habits healthy? Incorporating plenty of fruits and vegetables in your meal is important. Your plate should be filled with 75% vegetables and an even distribution of fruits and lean meats for the rest.

Eating less during dinner can also help your body digest excess fat effectively before you go to bed. If you really want to shed extra 10 pounds in two weeks, another important matter you must remember is to eat breakfast. This is still the most important meal of the day and effective in providing the energy you need to face the day ahead.

Stop Overeating and Lose As Much As 10 Pounds

Obesity is one of the leading causes of death. It can lead to various complications of the heart and the entire cardiovascular system. Hypertension, diabetes and even cancer can ramify from simply being overweight. The mere fact is that obesity can be fought with simple measures. There are even those who managed to lose weight simply by cutting back on their food consumption and learning how to stop overeating.

Although this can obviously be easier said than done, overeating is conquerable with the right attitude and knowledge. Exploring the several ways to help you fight one of the most common causes of weight gain can definitely provide long term benefits.

Lessen Your Stress

Stress is on the top list of the causes of overindulging. Many individuals find it easier to forget their problems by indulging on huge amounts of food. Sometimes they even fail to notice just how much they are eating. Stress can definitely alter one's behaviour and causes uncontrollable manias and unhealthy habits.

There are even cases wherein sleepwalking – most of the time caused by stress – results in weight gain since sufferers don't know that they are eating while sleeping. This is truly horrific indeed and can further cause more serious health problems. To avoid this, try to find ways to lessen your stress.

Take some time off to be with yourself and for relaxation.

Love More by Eating Less

Everyone likes food but the majority loves it. Loving food so much that it causes you to always gain weight is a sign of excessiveness. Food consumption can be lessened without causing you to love it less. The basic key here is to eat in moderation. This is probably an age old technique but it still does the trick. Never forget to buy only the right quantity if you are buying food only for yourself.

Eat Before Going to a Party

During the old days, young women are advised to eat before going to a party so as not to embarrass themselves and avoid 'accidents'. Well, this is still true nowadays though carries additional perks. It is often when people forget to control themselves – most importantly their appetite – during a party.

It is hard to notice that you are already eating too much when you are socializing and rapt with excitement. Get your stomach full or half-full before going to a party to avoid overeating. Don't stand around the buffet table if you get easily tempted with food. Be a complete butterfly and 'flutter' around the party while mingling with your friends.

Know Your Calories

Knowing just how much calories you need to take everyday can help you manage and lost weight. There are several online sources that enable you to calculate this by taking your gender, height, age, current weight and daily activities into consideration. This can definitely help you become more aware of the food you eat once you know your daily recommended calorie intake.

Don't just take everything you need the next time you do your groceries. Look at the label and see if the items have a detailed nutritional facts printed. It is helpful to be conscious of how much calories you consume each day. Furthermore, this attitude can definitely help you stop overeating and even make you lose weight in the long run.

Techniques to Lose More Than 10 Pounds Healthily

Losing weight, if done correctly, can ultimately benefit you in the long run. Proper weight management can provide you with a number of advantages like a defence against chronic and harmful diseases, boost in self-esteem and more. However, you can't get a hold of these benefits if you lose weight unhealthily. It is extremely important not to go down that road if you want to lose more than 10 pounds healthily.

Adverse Effects of Improper Dieting

For most of us, especially those who are overweight, it is extremely hard to lose weight let alone dieting. Doing a complete 180 in terms of the way you eat requires strong will and an indomitable spirit to succeed and achieve a goal. Unfortunately, this can't be said true to all dieters.

Most of us don't realize that the improper ways or usage of dietary techniques can cause adverse effects to both the mind and the body. Major bodily systems can be damaged as well as mental behavior. For starters, eating disorders can be the ultimate outcome of improper dieting. Anorexia and bulimia are fairly common nowadays due to unhealthy dietary techniques. Though these achieve desired results, the effects are detrimental to the body and sometimes even cause death.

Why Water is Important to the Diet

Increasing water intake is an integral part of any type of dietary technique. It is one of the most important aspects of weight loss. Water and other liquids are capable of flushing the toxins and other excess elements out of the body. In short, regular and increased fluid intake during diet can help cleanse the body.

Sometimes when you eat foods containing excessive fat, the extra fats unused by the body is deposited into the muscles. Overtime, this can cause build up of fatty muscles instead of lean ones. Water, on the other hand, can definitely help the body get rid of some of these excess fats.

The Role of Metabolism in Losing Weight

Aside from liquids, metabolism also plays an important role in metabolism. Simply put, metabolism is the term used for the body's mechanism in burning daily calorie intake. There are several kinds of diets that harness the power of metabolism. Almost all dieting methods aim at improving and increasing the body's metabolic rate. This is for the simplest reason that the faster the body's metabolic rate, the faster it is to burn calories.

Conversely, a slow metabolic rate can cause heavily build of fats in the body. You can help your body's metabolic rate in two simple ways: by exercising regularly and limiting your daily calorie intake.

The Benefits of Vegetables and Fruits

Another extremely important and probably the basic requirement of dieting are fruits and vegetables. These two types of food are very crucial in helping the body lose and manage weight. For starters, fruits contain natural sugar, some even fibres, that can help the body's energy level and bowel movements. Drinking fresh fruit juices is one way of helping the body lose weight faster.

Furthermore, vegetables contain dietary fibres helpful in flushing out toxins. In the simplest terms, fibre enriched vegetables cannot be digested and therefore always expelled from the body. When they are expelled, they tend to carry with them toxins and excess fat deposits. Eating such types of foods can definitely help you lose more than 10 pounds healthily and successfully.

The Diet Plans to Help You Lose 10 Pounds

You can jumpstart your quest for weight loss with an effective diet plan. There are plenty of diet plans to help you lose 10 pounds and more available virtually everywhere: from television ads to magazines to the Internet. Most of the diet plants are even designed to help you target problematic areas of the body. Of course, there are still several factors involved in the process of weight loss. Losing weight doesn't even compare to maintaining and gaining. That is why a proper mind set is important.

The High Protein Diet

One example of an effective dietary plan is the high protein diet. Protein is effective in building healthy muscles. We all know that carbohydrates and fats can effectively satiate a person but protein is even more effective. Recent studies now show that a certain component of protein has the ability to affect satiety. People under a high protein diet apparently experience an improvement in satisfaction, decrease in hunger and eventual weight loss, which is fairly significant.

This type of diet involves reducing fat consumption for up to 20% while increasing protein by 30%. The remaining 50% is for the carbohydrates, which is still essential in helping the body perform daily tasks. Combining this diet with a decrease in the daily calorie intake can improve results considerably.

The High Fibre Diet

Aside from a high protein diet, one dietary plan that has been around for a very long time is the high fibre diet. Fibre has been known to provide several health benefits. When used in the diet, it can help in improving digestion and losing weight. There are two types of dietary fibre: the insoluble and soluble fibre.

The soluble fibre forms a gel-like substance when digested while the insoluble one helps in developing the bowel movement. Dietary fibre has the ability to slow the movement of food in the intestine thus allowing for proper nutrient absorption and causing prolonged satiety. Furthermore, fibre can even reduce the number of calories the body consumes from the ingested food.

Before Going on a Diet

Before undergoing any type of diet, it is important to consider several factors. Firstly, you should completely set your mind on success. Knowing the many benefits of weight loss can definitely help you commit on the process.

It is also important to check with your doctor before going on any specific weight loss program. This can help you identify the possible risks the diet can eventually cause. For instance, the high protein diet can be quite harmful if you have any liver and kidney problems. Knowing any pre-existing illnesses you have can help you identify the right type of diet for you.

Find a Buddy or a Group

A successful dieter is surrounded by supportive loved ones. Find a weight loss group in your neighbourhood to help you manage the fight against obesity. This is one of the most important parts of any diet plans to help you lose 10 pounds or even more effectively. An online weight loss buddy is also an effective way to help you succeed in your quest.

Remember that this type of change in your lifestyle can be stressful and you definitely need people

close to you around to keep you strong and
motivated.

The Fastest Ways to Lose 10 Pounds

Losing weight can sometime become a burden.
Whether you are pressured socially or internally,
weight loss is very hard to do without the proper
motivation. One of the basic and fastest ways to
lose 10 pounds or more is to set realistic goals
fueled by a purpose or reason.

Your purpose helps you become directed to a
singular goal – weight loss. Of course, your raison
d'etre for weight loss should be realistic and
personal. Losing weight just because you want to
impress someone you like can never help you
achieve your goal. Instead, why not make your
purpose entirely for your personal growth and
overall wellbeing?

The Basics of Losing Weight

Each kinds of weight loss program shares the same
fundamentals. Firstly, you must consume lesser
calories than you normally do. Secondly, you must
learn how to burn these calories for effective weight
loss. These can be easier said than done. However,
always remember that these obstacles are not
without their own solutions.

That is why experts are continuously looking for ways to make your weight loss journey an easy ride. However for now, you should settle for the traditional exercising and dieting. The only thing you need to do is to make your mission more worthwhile in your own way.

Indulge Yourself Once a Week

One of the challenges you must face when losing weight is the feeling of depravation. To answer this, you must remember to indulge once a week – have a cheat day! Many dieters find it especially helpful to lose weight knowing that they can still enjoy their favourite foods. However, a cheat day is different from a binge eating day. There is a thin line between indulging and excessiveness.

On the brighter side, there are several kinds of food that are considerably low in calories if consumed in moderation. For instance, enjoying daily fresh fruit salad with two ounces of whipped cream once a week only adds eight calories. If you like crustaceans so much but are afraid about the calorie content, you would be happy to know that 11 large pieces of shrimps only have 60 calories and 83 calories for every three ounces of lobster. Explore and diversify your cheat day. Just make sure you indulge in moderation.

Drink Water Instead of Coffee

Every morning, people would normally seek out coffee to help through the day. This should not be the case if you are trying to lose weight. Instead of drinking coffee, eat whole grain cereals and other fibre enriched foods during breakfast. Partner these with plenty of glasses of water.

Throughout the day, you should drink water instead of juice, especially those commercial and packaged ones. These juices have artificial flavouring and additives in them that can hinder your weight loss program.

Choose Smaller Plates

Downsizing plates is the latest addition in the trend of healthier lifestyles. Several studies show that the less food you put in your plate, the less you will eat. Regardless of how hungry you may be, putting too much food in your plate can cause you to eat more. The main concept of this technique is to trick the brain in thinking that you actually have in front of you a plate full of food. In reality you only have a smaller plate, which lessens the empty spaces on the plate fairly common on larger plates.

This is surely one of the fastest ways to lose 10 pounds or more in a matter of weeks.

Tips in Melting 10 Pounds in a Month

Melting 10 pounds in a month is probably the easiest and safest way to do for someone who is always on the go. If you are the type of person who is constantly busy with work, appointments and others, the last thing you need to do is lose weight. However, losing weight is still beneficial with regards to your everyday duties. Staying in shape can help you do your tasks faster and more efficiently. You have a vast amount of energy resource to help you survive a busy day at work.

First Step

One of the main requirements of losing weight is to decrease your daily calorie consumption. Normally, a month-long weight loss program requires you to cut as much as 600 to your calorie intake. The ratio of fat to protein to carbohydrates is also dependent on the calorie intake. As a result, your food intake will be dramatically decrease by up to 20%. Don't be frightened by these numbers since you are not depriving your body of anything. You are merely making an improvement.

Sweating is also another thing that you should change. You must increase the frequency you sweat everyday since sweating is a sign of burning calories. The most effective way to sweat is to perform some cardio exercises or aerobics. This can help your endurance and major bodily systems, i.e. respiratory and circulatory.

Second Step

The next step is to plan a gym schedule that would work for you. Going to the gym for at least thrice a week can help boost your weight loss. On the other hand, you can still exercise at home if in case you can't commit on a gym program due to busy schedules.

Purchase a pair of light dumbbells to help you get started. Perform weight-lifting everyday for at least 30 minutes and gradually increase according to your preference. The basic and most useful way to balance the exercises is to do a 30-minute cardio and 30-minute strength training routine daily. This wouldn't eat too much of your time since it can be done nearly any time of the day.

Third Step

This is the probably the hardest part of your weight loss regimen – diet. Eating a low-calorie diet rich with fibre and lean meats is advised. Stay away from trans-fat normally found on junk foods and especially French fries. Good for you if you rarely eat out since you can definitely monitor your food effectively if you always eat at home.

However, simply limiting the time and frequency one spends to eat dine out can help promote weight loss. Reduce or even eliminate fat from your diet and opt for baking, steaming or even raw with regards to the food you eat.

After One Month

You can definitely see the results of this diet after a month. Furthermore, you would be able to lose as much as one pound per day if you follow a strict exercise and dietary program. However, achieving the results would not mean cessation of the routine. Melting 10 pounds in one month can be a breeze but if you let it be after that period, you would find yourself gaining the lost weight.

Avoid this by continuing with your healthy routine or finding a regimen that can help you maintain your current figure.

Tips on How to Lose 10 Pounds in a Span of 6 Days

Weight loss programs that promise to deliver desired results in a matter of days might be too good to be true – it is not though. Shedding of a few extra pounds in the shortest period of time is doable but extremely difficult. Without the right knowledge and tools, you are sure to put a tremendous amount of damage on the body especially if you are trying to lose pounds in a span of 6 days.

Benefits of Intense Dieting

A diet aimed at improving one's eating habits is absolutely beneficial in terms of losing weight. If done right, it can produce desired results even in the shortest amount of time. If you want to lose weight in less than a week, it is advisable to perform a three-day intense dieting. This only means a total overhaul of your eating habits.

Be ready to clean your fridge of unhealthy foods and stock it with healthier ones. Get rid of junk foods on your cabinets and instead look for healthier alternatives, which you can munch on whenever you experience cravings. There are several diets that can produce intense results though they require you to adapt to extreme eating habits. Fasting or lessening the food you eat is one way of intense dieting. This type of diet requires you to lessen your portions every meal and eat only the right kinds of food. Though there are plenty of other diets out there, a fast diet is extremely effective.

More than Just an Exercise

Intense dieting should be partnered with the right type of exercise regimen. Exercise can also be beneficial in terms of helping you in your diet. Going camping is one way to help you in your diet while allowing you to perform intense exercise at the same time. If you plan to go on a three to six day of fast dieting, going camping for the same time length is very helpful. Camping will keep you away from eating excessively and unhealthy types of food.

Advantages of Master Cleanse

The Master Cleanse Diet is another intense type of dieting. It has been around of nearly fifty years and yet continues to be popular. The main advantages of Master Cleanse diet is probably rejuvenation and speedy weight loss. In addition, this type of diet can help you fight certain types of health problems you might be suffering from.

Other benefits of the Master Cleanse Diet are youthfulness, detoxification, boost in energy level, and ease from body pains. However before even thinking about undergoing such type of diet, you must realize that the Master Cleanse diet is extreme and very intense. Unlike any diet wherein most people sail through easily, not many people can last one day of Master Cleanse Diet. On the good side though, the Master Cleanse can be doable with the right methods.

Master Cleanse In A Nutshell

The Master Cleanse Diet requires a concoction of specific lemonade. The drink normally consists of: 2 tbsp. organic maple syrup, 2 tbsp. organic lemon juice, 10 oz. of water and a pinch of cayenne pepper. This recipe is designed for a single glass. If you are undergoing this type of diet, you must prepare six to twelve servings of the mixture.

If you want to lose 10 pounds in a span of 6 days or even less, you must only drink the lemonade whenever you are hungry and during mealtime. Deviating will render the diet useless.

Tips to Help You Lose 10 Pounds in 6 Weeks

Most of the time, due to inability to commit to a certain diet and exercise regimen, people fail to lose even the slightest significant weight loss in a period of one month. Furthermore, gaining back the lost weight usually occurs if one cannot continue with the commitment to diet. The only solution to this is to increase the time frame for the weight loss journey.

The common cause of failure is work. People who are too busy to lose weight must not commit in the first place lest risking the so-called yo-yo diet. Fortunately, there is a weight loss program that can be easily done by the busiest of people.

Tip No. 1

For your breakfast always opt for one serving of cereal rather than a full English breakfast. The best thing to do when trying to lose weight is to cut the amount of calories you take. A traditional serving of cereal for most people is actually equivalent to two servings. What you should do is to get that measuring cup ready and accurately measure your breakfast cereals: three-fourths to one cup or depending on the label of the cereal.

Tip No. 2

Choose steam and even raw for butter and margarine. Although French cuisine is definitely mouth-watering, butter is an absolute no-no during diets. The same goes for margarine. Steamed vegetables are healthier than those sautéed in butter.

On the other hand, you can still significantly lower your butter and margarine consumption if you cannot completely erase it from your healthy must-eat list. A decrease of one tablespoon of butter everyday can save you more than 4,000 calories, which is enough to help you lose pounds in six weeks.

Tip No. 3

The best way to lose weight is to skip your routine late night snacks. It easier for the body to gain weight at night since the extra calories are stored and turned to fats instead of burnt. Try to limit your nightly snacks to 150 calories and choose those guilt-free dietary snacks.

You can even choose to drink a tea instead of coffee before bed to kill the craving. You would save as much as 11,000 calories in the course of six weeks, which means a three-pound weight loss.

Tip No. 4

It is healthier to eat a sandwich for lunch instead of a full lunch meal. However, make sure that you skip the mayonnaise and cheese on your sandwich. These two packs a lot of calories that require some time to burn. Instead of putting cheese or mayonnaise, opt for mustard, which contains a healthier five calories per teaspoon. If you have the habit of eating a piece of sandwich everyday, you would be able to save up to 8,800 calories – a two and a half pounds weight loss.

Tip No. 5

Always be mindful of the extra calories you consume sometimes unconsciously. Most people don't realize that the number one contributing factor in weight gain is the habit of taking small bites from others' meals. For instance, you would surely help your weight loss journey if you eliminate your habit of taking home an extra packet of salad dressing or ketchup from the restaurant or taking a small bite from a friend's dessert.

These tips are designed to help you create a healthier lifestyle free of unwanted excess calories. These are guidelines that can help you achieve a healthier you. More so, doing all these tips regularly can eventually help you lose 10 pounds in six weeks.

Weight Loss Menu Plans for Shedding Off That Extra 10 Pounds

Dieting without the knowing the right dish to cook is like finding something in a very dark place. Mistakes can be easily made without proper guidance. That is why there are numerous of weight loss menu plans that can last for weeks to help you get things going with your diet. These dishes are intended to help you lost weight by providing low calories.

Breakfast Dishes

The most important meal of the day should be packed with energy boosting meals. It is crucial to make yourself full during breakfast to help you get through the entire day. One example of a healthy breakfast meal is one split of toasted English muffin topped with any type of cheese. Broil the muffin until the cheese melts. You can partner the muffin with half a grapefruit and a dash of brown sugar.

If you want a fiber enriched breakfast, grab one and one-fourth cups of your bran flake cereal and add a cup of fat-free milk to it. Top the cereal with potassium-rich banana to make it tastier.

Lunch Dishes

Spinach salad is a very healthy lunch dish. Create this dish by topping three to four cups of baby spinach with a piece of sliced hard-boiled egg. In addition, you can add crumbled bacon strips, five pieces of thinly sliced mushrooms, a third of a cup of croutons, three slices of red onion and one-fourth cup of feta cheese. Toss the ingredients together and drizzle with your favorite dressing preferably a balsamic vinegar and olive oil.

If you want a simpler meal during lunch, a sandwich is perfect. A simple raisin bread sandwich with organic peanut butter and honey should help you get through to dinner. Couple this sandwich with a refreshing cup of fat-free milk.

Dinner Dishes

It is very important to eat a light meal during dinner. One perfect example of a healthy dinner meal is the Savory Asian Patty, which you can easily store in the freezer. The ingredients of the dish are:

• One pound turkey breast
• Eight pieces of diced water chestnuts
• Two garlic cloves, minced
• Four pieces of thinly sliced onions
• Half a cup of unsweetened applesauce
• Four tablespoons of soy sauce.

Proceed by mixing all the ingredients together and making four patties. You only need one of the patties so you better save the three for later. Coat a nonstick skillet with cooking spray and cook the patty over medium heat. Make sure that both sides of the patty are cooked thoroughly.

Serve the patty with three-fourths cup of brown rice, a teaspoon of rice vinegar and soy sauce and half a teaspoon of sesame oil. Furthermore, you can add two cups of steamed broccoli and a cup of berries to make it a complete meal.

In-Between Meals

Cravings are particularly hard to control when you are not used to dieting. Changing the way you eat is probably one of the hardest parts of losing weight. Remember that you don't have to starve yourself during any kind of diet. Eat a snack in case your cravings start to help you through the day. However, keep in mind to make your snacks healthy. For instance, instead on munching on chocolate chip cookies, opt of soaked almonds or fat-free yogurt.

Other important parts of some of the weight loss menu plans are multivitamin and mineral supplements. Taking 250 to 400 milligrams of calcium daily is recommended since you are most likely not going to get enough of it by slashing your food consumption substantially.

USEFUL LINKS

Lose Weight-NHS
http://www.nhs.uk/LiveWell/loseweight/Pages/Loseweighthome.aspx

Holland and Barrett
http://www.hollandandbarrett.com/pages/categories.asp?cid=246

Weight Loss Resources
http://www.weightlossresources.co.uk/calories/burning_calories/burn_more_calories.htm

Sainsburys Diets
http://www.sainsburysdiets.co.uk/

Slimming World
http://www.slimmingworld.com/

The Simple Guide
To
Pet Adoption

By
Warren Brown

INTRODUCTION

Dear Reader,

Thank you for selecting this book about Pet Adoption. I do hope that this book helps you to decide to adopt a pet. Give a pet a home today and make the world a better place to live.

Warm Regards

Warren Brown
London
2012

This book will help you to...

1. Look at having your own Pet
2. Think about Pets without a home.
3. Help you to decide on the best way to go about Adopting a Pet of your own.
4. Realize that you can make a difference in the life of an animal which needs a home.
5. Look at the pros and cons of pet adoption.
6. Create a plan of action to adopt a pet.
7. Look at all the alternatives available to you for pet adoption.
8. Help you to do more research into the field of pet adoption.
9. Assist in guiding you to making your decision.
10. Give a Pet a Home Today!

Safe Haven: Why Pets are Put Up for Adoption

There are so many pets that are homeless nowadays. According to the Humane Society of the United States, an estimated 8 to 10 million cats and dogs enter animal shelters yearly. Meanwhile a terrifying number of 4 to 5 million cats and dogs are being euthanized by shelters. The reason? Because there are not enough people going to shelters for pet adoption.

These figures do not include those in small, local and home-based shelters. There are also animal rescue organizations that take abused and abandoned animals. There are also hundred of animals left to stray in the streets.

Pets end up in shelters due to numerous reasons. There are pets that are abused and hurt by their owners thinking that this is another form of training and discipline among their pets. Animals victims of these extreme cased can be rescued and if the animals are not showing any behavioural problems, may be put up for adoption.

Another reason why there are so many animals in shelters is because there are more and more animals straying or roaming around. There are guardians who let their pets roam outside their premises and never bother to look for them once they are gone. Also these animals do not have any identification tags. That is why it is difficult to return them to their owners.

The most common reason that an animal shelter can hear from pet parents surrendering their pets is that they are moving. There are guardians who do not want to pay to transport their pets, guardians moving to apartments not allowing pets inside, guardians who do not want to pay a pet deposit, and many more. It is important to remember that pets are not old pieces of furniture that can be left behind just because you can buy another one. Pets are living things that have repaid us with loyalty and devotion.

Having a baby is another reason why pet parent give up their pets for adoption. SPOT (Stopping Pet Overpopulation Society, Inc), an alliance of animal lovers, dog/cats rescuers and veterinarians in Atlanta, recommends that people have their family first then adopt a pet. If it is not possible, then it is best to pick a breed or mixed bred that is known to be good with children.

It is important to remember before getting a pet that they require attention, time and money. There are pet parents surrendering their pets because they can no longer provide time to take care of them. Also others may find it too expensive to raise and take care of a pet. It is important to think that taking care of pets is a commitment that you are ready to take and be responsible for the next 10 to 15 years.

Behavioural problems of pets is also another reason for giving up a pet. Too much barking, chewing everything, too hyper or aggressiveness of the pet are the common cited behavioural problems cited. Of course, dogs who do not undergo obedience training will be rambunctious and wild. Dogs who do not socialize much will be aggressive against other animals and even to other people.

It is important for a parent to get a pet, only if, the parent wants it as much as the children want the animal. When children lose interest in the pet, it is more likely that the unfortunate animal will be given up for adoption. It is important to always ask yourself, as a parent before getting a pet the real reason for getting one.

There are also incidents that elderly guardians could no longer take care of their pets because of death or they would have to go to a nursing facility. If the pet parent is already a senior citizen it is important to take into consideration the age of the pet and who will take care of it when the situation turns worse. If it is uncertain who will take care of the pet, it is best to adopt a pet that is already and wonderfully housebroken older dog.

There are many reasons why pets are put up for adoption almost every day. It might be unfortunate events that happened to the pet parent or just avoidance of responsibility. It is important whenever we are getting a pet to consider if we are indeed ready for it and committed in taking care of it.

Behind the Scenes: What is Pet Adoption?

Pet adoption is the process of taking responsibility for a pet or animal. The pet or animal may have been abandoned or surrendered to a shelter because their owners are unable to care for them.

Common places where you can adopt a pet would be in animal shelters (for dogs, it is more known as dog pound). Pets that are in captivity without any identification and unclaimed by the owner are also adoptable pets. There are also people who put up advertisements putting their pet into adoption. Aside from this, the internet is a good source of adoptable pets. There are several websites that displays information, photos about adoptable pets.

Irresponsible owners, owners who abuse their animals continuously, may lose their pets altogether. There are animal rescue groups that save animals from abusive and violent owners. Not only animal rescue groups or organizations respond to calls of abused animals, but also they take abandoned, unwanted and stray pets. Rescue groups are frequently run by volunteers.

Pet adoption from rescue groups most of the times has stricter or more rigid process. Most of the times, it would include veterinary reference, background check and conducting a home visit. There would be adoption fees but these do not cover transportation for picking up the pet, providing veterinary care, vaccinations, training and food.

It is important for most rescue organizations to do these since pet adoption really is about knowing if the new owners of the pet will be able to handle the responsibility and care of their new pet. This is to avoid that the same thing happen again to the unfortunate animal.

Animal shelters on the other hand, are run by the government. However, animal shelters are the best place for pet adoption. Not only do they have adult animals, they also have kittens and puppies. An interesting fact about an animal shelter is that about 25 to 30 per cent of animals in the shelters are purebreds.

Animal shelters also follow necessary procedures to ensure the proper care of animals put up for adoption. Many shelters offer adoption counselling and follow up assistance. This process serves as a background check on the persons who will adopt but also an effort to provide good matches between people and animals.

Animal shelters also do require adoption fees. But adoption fees are much less than the animal's purchase price in the pet store. Another benefit from adopting from shelters is that the pet is more likely to be already vaccinated, dewormed and spayed or neutered.

Even so, the new owner, most of the times, still encounter some challenges with the pet. These cases happen mostly with animals who are victims of abuse and neglect. The new owners should always provide extra patience in understanding and training the animals. These will help the pets to overcome the past.

According to Kelly Connolly of the Humane Society of the United States, there is an estimated 6 to 8 million dogs and cats enter shelters each year. With these big numbers, there are just an estimated 3,500 standing animal shelters in the United State, not including an unknown number of smaller, local and home-based rescue organizations. These figures only show that there are not enough places that could accommodate our pets.

For people who are interested in having pets, pet adoption is a great way of saving money. At the same time provide a life-long home and love for animals in shelters and rescue groups.

An Overview about How a Pet Adoption Centre Works

What do you do if you want to adopt pets? There are actually many options for you these days if you are pondering about such thing. Your main consideration must be to look for the right pet adoption centre where you will get the animal that can change your life forever.

Big Responsibility

Owning a pet is indeed a big responsibility. As much as these pets bring laughter and fun to your household, it cannot be helped that they may also cause distractions and destruction. And why is that? They are animals. And as much as you train them, their instincts are not the same from yours. So you must not expect them to follow everything that you say with compliance and retention that you can get from a child.

So think hard about your decision before you settle on anything that may affect your life as well as that of the animals. You must choose the pet that will suit your lifestyle the best. If you have acquired an animal, you must do everything in your capacity to prove that you are its rightful owner.

Emotionally, you must be attached to your pets. This will help in instances wherein you don't like what they have done or have caused you. You will not instantly get mad at them enough to throw them out because of the connection that you are sharing with your pet. Physically, you must only choose the kind of pets that you can keep up with. If you don't have enough time to spare for a pet, you can settle for the tamer types and those that will not require you to get involved in activities with them. And of course, financially, you must be ready to pay for any medical conditions that your pet may need in instances that they get sick or get entangled into accidents.

Adoption Centre

The centres for the adoption of pets are being built by organizations that are concerned about the welfare of animals. They aim to help the animals, give them temporary shelter while providing them their basic necessities like food and warmth. Their goal is to give these animals the rightful owners who will take care of them.

These shelters bring in different animals that have varied backgrounds. Some were abused, many are neglected and there are those that are lost. There are also some animals that are handicapped and were left at the shelters by their owners who couldn't care for them given the situation.

The shelter, as much as possible, will go out of their way to find sponsors for their organizations. They give the animals on their care the proper medication, vaccination and treatment for these pets to remain healthy while at their care. Some of the shelters will require you some fees when you adopt an animal. But this is still less expensive than buying a pet from a commercial store. In most cases, you will be assisted by the people at such centres to find the perfect pet that will fit the kind of life that you are leading. They will lead you to the animal that they are sure that you can handle given your situation.

You can browse through the Internet to find a pet adoption centre near you. You can also ask for help at your local vets. You can also ask suggestions from the pet stores or some people who may have already used the service of such centres.

An Analysis on the Best Times to Try Pet Adoption

If you are set about owning a pet, it may be better if you will first inquire about the best times to do pet adoption. Inquiries are a must if you want to get what you want and what will fit in to the kind of life that you are leading.

Not because you want a very big dog are you going to be allowed by adoption centers to have one. The centers will do a lifestyle check to find out if what you want is really what you need. The match should be right. You cannot get an active pup if you don't have time to play with it or take time to do rounds of running with the pet each day.

Who you are will determine what kind of pet you deserve. Being a pet owner is a big responsibility. The animal shelter will do their best to make sure that the decision will be beneficial for you and your chosen pet.

The Costs

This is one factor that you must be prepared for. Acquiring a pet through adoption is less costly than when you buy them on commercial pet stores. But there are some considerations that you must also be prepared to allot for. This includes, most importantly, is the medical needs of your pets. You should be ready that just like you, they may get sick from time to time. And the sickness may vary from simple to severe. And accidents may also happen when you least expect it so you have to have that extra budget to be able to handle the situation.

Save a Life

If you are still undecided about adopting a pet, here is one great motivation for you. Did you know that every year, more than four million of companion animals are being destroyed in the United States alone? So in your decision to adopt a pet, you are also saving a life in the process.

If you have no idea how to start the process of adoption, you can look for your local center or the one nearest you of the Humane Association of the United States. You can also ask the help of the veterinarians near you and they can point you to the right people. You can also do the inquiries at the pet stores in your locality. But please be sure that before you precede any further with the adoption process that you are ready in all aspects that may require you to be.

Finance is a priority. But aside from that, you must also be ready to open up emotionally. Animals are like humans, they need to feel loved and taken cared for. You must also talk about your decision to the important people of your life who will also be interacting with the pet. This is a serious matter that requires you to be responsible for your every decision.

The Right Time
The best times to do pet adoption, of course, is when you are ready in all aspect mentioned above. But if you want to get the best deals, it will be best for you to seek out the shelters in springtime and early fall. These are the breeding seasons so your choices will be a lot varied.

Meanwhile, if you don't want to be stuck with minimal choices, do not go during Christmas season. Many people are adopting during this time and so the process is being hurried.

An Overview of the Costs of Pet Adoption

You can know the costs of pet adoption before you commit to it. The easiest option may be to open your PC and connect to the World Wide Web. You must remember that your choice of animals will depend a lot on the lifestyle that you are leading. Adoption centers can help you with the process of finding the right one for you. They are also concerned about the well-being of the animals after they have left the center. So as much as possible, they want the right pets to land on the right hands.

Does it already sound like a dating game wherein people are being matched according to their traits and preferences? Well, that is very much true. As the pet owner, you must also make sure that when you already acquired the animal, you must do everything in your capacity to look out for its well-being. Now it is already sounding more like parenting, right? But this shouldn't scare you. Pets bring lots of joy for those who are open to accept them with loving arms.

But before your thoughts go as far as the many advantages of being a pet owner, you must first be informed about the costs that it would take for you to find the right pet.

1. In calculating the annual costs of owning a pet through adoption, the American Society for the Prevention of Cruelty to Animals suggests that the following items must be included: food, treats, toys, required licensing if any, medical treatment and vaccinations. They have come up with the following figures for the pets listed below.

• Fish will cost about $20. The aquarium's prices differ from $20 to $200 and even higher depending on the quality and the features.

• The prices of dogs will differ depending on the size and breed. A medium built may cost about $600 while a large built can be up to $800.

• Rabbits are easy to deal with. But the costs for this type can be up to $700.

• Cats may be within the range of $500 to $600.

• The prices of birds will also depend on the size and type. A small one can cost about $100 to $150.

After you have acquired these pets, it is your responsibility to provide for their shelter, fun and training if you want. You may want to purchase cages for your pets, training bundles and dog crates. The costs for these can range from $80 to $500.

2. You must also be prepared for unexpected conditions such as accidents and sudden medical problems. You must save up for your pets as well for you to be able to afford the treatments in such conditions.

3. To give you a detailed sample of the costs of adopting a pet, here's one example where you can base your decisions from. As stated previously, the annual costs that you may incur from owning a cat can reach from $500 to $600. And why is that? Here is the breakdown. The cost of adopting an adult cat is $60. The prices vary from location and the breed

of the feline that you choose. If you will buy cats from pet stores, the prices may range from $150 up to $1000. The cats from the center have been neutered ($30 up to $80) or spayed ($45 to $90). The vaccinations for its first year can be about $150 to $300. Cats must also undergo FELV or Feline Aids and FELV or Feline Leukemia testing that can be about $50 to $80 per test.

But the costs of pet adoption must not discourage you from being a pet owner. The joys your pets will add to your life will make it all worthwhile.

Easy Steps towards Virtual Pet Adoption

Do you have a website for your business? Or do you maintain a blog for personal purposes? Or you may not have any of these but you are an avid Internet user. Then you may find the idea of virtual pet adoption as something interesting.

The Idea
The notion behind this all is that you, as the Internet user, will have to go to certain URL address known as the virtual pet adoption center. From that site, you can adopt a pet of your choice for free. Where that virtual pet will go? You can display it on your website or you can just bookmark the page where you want it to be.

Are you getting the idea? This is like teaching a virtual pet owner to care for something that will in turn make them happy, just like what real pets do to you. This makes your cyber experience more fun and enjoyable because you have the pet to look forward to whenever you open your PC and you go online.

How to Get One
The process is simple. You can look over any search engines for the popular websites that offer this tool. Be careful with the sites. Make sure that they pass all the anti-virus and spam filtering settings of your connection. When you visit these sites, read the instructions carefully. Make sure that the pets are safe to be downloaded, if this can be done.

Choose the animal that you'd want to be your virtual pet. There are a lot of choices actually. The popular ones include puppy, penguin, cat, spider, pig, fish, hamster, a duck and so on. The list can actually accommodate all your preferences when it comes to this. Then after choosing the animal, you must name your pet. What do you want to call it? And then you will choose what colour is your pet going to be. You will be given a code that you can copy and paste on the space provided for such on your own website. This kind of entertainment comes for free.

How Does It Work?
Once installed, you will the master of your chosen pet. They will follow your mouse on every direction. Other tricks that some of them can do include the following. The spider will spin webs on your screen while you are watching it. You can feed the fish by clicking your PC's mouse. The penguin

will make you feel light as it sits on the iceberg and moves around. It loses balance and falls into the cold water. The tiger will wave back and purrs at you. The puppy will bark at you until you give them treats. The bunny hops around while you are clicking on it.

Your website or the page that you have bookmarked will become home to your chosen pet. It will also add to its appeal and may increase traffic to your site. Just remember that just like in the real sense of acquiring a pet, having an online pet will require you to look out for it whenever you are online. Do this for fun and enjoyment. Just make sure to instill the good values that you will be able to pick up along the process.

You see, virtual pet adoption is easy. It will make your website come alive. It will also make you feel happier and relaxed whenever you are online.

Finding the Pet Adoption Portal for You

For many people, finding an appropriate pet adoption portal is the only thing that stands in the way of them getting a new pet. They are the type of people who already want to get pets, love pets, want to get ready for caring for a pet if they aren't already, and are only looking for ways to get access to the pets they want to give homes to.

For those who are not keen on buying their pets from the pet store, their options for getting pets are threefold: through rescue organizations, through pet shelters, and through the internet.

Rescue organizations are run by volunteers who want to save pets from the threats they face when they are left to roam and fend for themselves in the cities. These rescue organizations aim to cut down on the near 70% of animals that get killed yearly due to harsh conditions and overpopulation. These rescue organizations help nurse these dogs and cats back to life, and help find suitable homes that will adopt them. Their team of expert volunteers and counsellors offer both compatibility assessment and adoption counselling to help facilitate the entire process.

These rescue organizations, because they prefer to be able to save as many animals as possible, would prefer individuals to return the pets they adopted if, for any reason, they feel it is not the right pet for them. Communicating your expectations clearly to the volunteers at the organization may help narrow the search for your perfect dog. These rescue organizations are home to about 21 to 30% purebreds each year, making them equally attractive places to search pets from.

Animal shelters provide the same sort of service to rescue organizations, because they want to provide animals all the care and support they need to survive. There are a huge number of animal shelters in existence, so it's important to check whether the shelter you are approaching is good or bad. Good shelters provide animals with a clean, sanitary environment, and captivity conditions that will not constrict reasonable movement where they are kept. Some animal shelters also recommend that you get a pet that has already been previously sterilized.

This is to avoid instances when individuals want only one pet, and end up having one pet with 5 to 7 offspring. Shelters want to be able to get pets to care for off their hands and into better homes, and giving one for adoption in return for having to accept the 5 or 7 offspring it will be have is not commensurate. Ask about mandatory sterilization and whether it's recommended for your pet. However, if you intend to grow a pet and it's young ones through generations in the family, inform the shelter that you do not wish the pet sterilized before it is released to you.

The last portal you can make use of is the internet. With the advent of the growing consumer awareness through online information channels, the internet has made it easier to disseminate information and provide access to the same. There are websites online exclusively designed to accommodate those who wish to adopt pets.

The mechanism that is underlying the entire system is that the website accepts only listings for pets open for adoption and not any other listing. This helps keep the message that the facility is only to help make adoptions possible.

This pet adoption portal may prove to be effective especially for those who have very little time in their hands to visit shelters by themselves.

How to Find Free Pet Adoption Websites

The best things in life are free. This song lyric is true in most instances. But do you actually envision free pet adoption? No, this is not the virtual pets that you can download and use at your websites. This is also free but the main difference lies in the pets that you will be getting. Forget the codes that you have to copy and paste on your site because this is the real thing. You can get real animals that can be your pets just by excavating through the available online adoption centers.

Make a Difference

Every year, about four million animals are being executed in the United States alone. Think about just how many more experience the same fate all over the world. But you cannot solely put the blame on the people who decide on these things. There are many pets that are being uncared for and as a result, these animals wander aimlessly. They experience the world's cruelty that is why they sometimes end up as cruel and can be harmful to other people.

Pet adoption can be achieved in many ways. There are centers wherein you can get the animals with a minimal fee. The costs that will be incurred in this process are still much lower than when you opt to buy the pets on commercial stores. You can gain information about such centers on your local vets and even on the pet stores on your locality. The advantage of this route is that you are assured that the animals that you are getting have been treated with proper vaccinations and other required treatments. Most of the time, you will be assisted by the facilitators of the center so that they can match you with the kind of pet that will suit your lifestyle. This way, you are assured that you will be getting not only what you want but also what you need.

In any adoption scenario though, it will be better to do this during the springtime or even in early fall. These are considered the breeding seasons. You will have many choices with the kinds and breeds of the animals on the shelters. Meanwhile, Christmastime is not a good season to complete the adoption. Many people are actually doing this during this month that you will have only minimal choices. And besides, with all hustles and the bustles that the occasion may present, you may even want to go a holiday trip, you can afford to worry about the pet that you will left behind at home.

Perfect timing is also a key to be successful with this venture. You have to find your perfect match in terms of pets. And you have to find it during when you can really allot time for it.

There are also free adoption centers available for you if this is the setup that you prefer. You can find the right leads mostly on websites. These kinds are being held up by non-profit organizations that aim to help lost animals to be found by their rightful owners. These are the people who would really care for them even if they don't look as superb as the ones available commercially or that they don't look as cute as a famous' personalities featured pet on TV.

Take time to browse the Net for the links that can guide you to free pet adoption websites. Think about any steps that you will take after you click on the sites. And before even setting your eyes on the pet that you want to adopt, make sure that you are really ready to welcome the animal into your home and into your life.

Looking for Free Pet Adoption Opportunities

Often, people who have never had pets before entertain the thought of having pets when the opportunity for free pet adoption arises. Those who entertain the possibility of using these free channels often do not request to get their own pets because they are confused as to how to go about the entire process. Luckily, there are a lot of adoption centres and shelters that can assist families and homeowners in their pursuit of the perfect pet.

One of the best places to look is a rescue organization. These rescue organizations for pets are part of a big effort in order to help save the almost 7 million pet dogs and cats that die due to the lack of care and overpopulation in the streets. Their goal is to keep these animals of the streets, and possibly, find for themselves a sustainable home to stay in for the rest of their lives.

With this goal in mind, these rescue organizations often try their best to make sure they are able to find the best possible home for the pets they have rescued. They do this firstly by making use of the services of volunteers. More than a strategy to cut costs, the use of volunteers in the facility helps them make sure that they know the pets they have very well and that these pets are well taken care of.

This is because volunteers at pet shelters and rescue organizations are often individuals who are very much interested in taking care of animals, and invest time and effort in getting to know animals in order to give them what they need. Because they know these animals so well, they are also able to know what sort of environment will best suit the pet once it is ready for adoption.

They also have a series of application steps and screening interviews for prospective adopters. This helps them assess the intention of the people seeking to adopt pets. Moreover, they are able to assess which pets may be most compatible with the people seeking pets to adopt. Through the series of interactions these volunteers have, they are able to cross-reference about the pets they've taken care of with the personality of the prospective owners.

Some of these individuals seeking to adopt pets can come into the facility already looking for particular breeds, or are more inclined to a pure-bred dog or cat over a mixed breed. What they may not expect, however, is that these rescue facilities can have a 30% population of purebreds at any given time. This, of course, is not to disparage the remaining 70% of the hybrids, who are equally wonderful as pets.

As they go through the entire application process, these rescue facilities often offer adoption counselling, which will allow the individual or family adopting to cope with the challenges of adjusting to a new pet. After all, they have to make sure that their current home and lifestyle conditions are conducive to giving love, attention, and care to a formerly unloved pet.

If, for some reason, some incompatibility results regardless of the preparation already put into place, these rescue organizations offer individuals the opportunity to return a pet. This is to help reduce the probability of pet owners simply leaving their pets out in the cold, or neglecting them because of an inherent dislike. At the end of the day, the goal of these rescue organizations is to keep these pets in safe homes, making an incompatibility compromise necessary.

At the end of the day, free pet adoption shouldn't scare people, especially with shelters offering as much assistance as they can along the way.

Online Pet Adoption – Looking After a Virtual Pet

Having a furry friend at home surely has its ups and downs. But did you know that there are these cute little critters called virtual pets that have become a craze in cyberspace these days? Online pet adoption sites allow you to select a pet to take care of. Virtual pets are one of the newest trends that never fail to fascinate both children and adults alike. They have become so popular with a lot of web users, investing time and emotions into their overall care and well-being.

You can select from a wide array of animals from dogs, cats, hamsters, pigs, monkeys, horses, snakes and many others. If you are looking for eccentric creatures to look after, there are also dragons, aliens and monsters available. The choices for a virtual pet to adopt are practically unlimited.

Jazzing up your personal sites

There are numerous sites which you can drop by and adopt a virtual pet. You can put them on your blogs to make them look more interesting. In fact, as much as most of these virtual pets come for free, they are also compatible to embed in most social networking sites of your choice.

Once you have registered with a virtual pet site, you can select the gender and the colour of your furry friend. Then you get to give it a name as well. A code will be generated for you to copy and paste wherever you wish your pet to appear on your personal website. You get to see your virtual pet and tend to their needs, like feeding and playing with it, whenever you log in to your site.

Teaching kids how to care for pets

What better way to train your kids in caring for pets than letting them experience having one virtually? These virtual pets are replicas of animals; they seek the same interaction from their owners essentially just like the real thing. Your kids will develop their sense of responsibility while looking after the pet of their choice, while having fun at the same time.

Unlike real animals, virtual pets will enable your kids to discover the enjoyment of having a pet without nearly as much maintenance as their real-life counterparts. The kids will discover how to attend to their pets' needs on their own, without their parents constantly reminding them to feed, bathe and walk their virtual furry pals. What will further motivate the kids to ensure the well-being of their virtual pets is the points they earn from it. The more points that they get, the more stuff they can purchase for their pets. They can buy them food, clothes, toys, houses and other items that will make the virtual pets happier.

Of course no virtual pet can give the kind of pleasure like only a real pet can give. But in the meantime, one can take on the satisfaction and enjoyment given by these cyber critters. It's experiencing having a pet, without the actual problems, which makes virtual pet adoption popular. Some of the great online pet adoption sites you may visit include:

* Bunnyhero Labs -
http://bunnyherolabs.com/adopt/
* Adopt Me - http://www.adoptme.com
* Perfect Petzzz - http://www.perfectpetzzz.com
* VirtualPups - http://www.virtualpups.com
* GiroPets - http://www.giropets.net
* Marapets - http://www.marapets.com
* Furry-Paws - http://www.furry-paws.com
* Fishland - http://www.fishland.com

Pet Adoption as the Solution

Pet adoption is taking responsibility over an animal that has been put up for adoption due to experience of abuse, violence, neglect and etc. with previous owners. With pet adoption, animals are given the chance in finding the appropriate, caring and life long home for them. Aside from this humane chance we are giving to man's best friend, there are also benefits from adopting animals.

The Humane Society of the United States estimates an whopping 8 to 10 million cats and dogs that enter shelters ever year. From these numbers, there is estimated 4 to 5 million of pets euthanized in shelters. Numbers of strays that die due to starvation are not included in this data.

With these sad figures, pet adoption is a great way of saving a life of a homeless animal. Animal euthanasia is being done because there are too many people giving up their pets and too few people adopting from shelters. There is limited space in shelters, euthanasia is a very hard decision to make by staff members to make way for new animals pouring into their doors.

Animals in shelter dying by euthanasia can be dramatically removed by adopting pets in shelters instead of buying them in pet stores. By adopting an animal from shelters, other animals can be saved and rescued else where and provided a home.

Animal shelters, unlike what pet adoption myths say, have healthy animals. Shelters often get as much information from previous owners to determine what kind of vaccination has already been provided. Aside from medical care investigation, shelters also provide the necessary vaccination and many spay o neuter the animals before being adopted.

Worrying about the temperament or behaviour of the animals is also not a big issue. Unlike the common misconception that animals are taken into shelters due to behaviour problems, personal reasons by the owner themselves are the most common factors.

Everybody knows that having pets have actual benefits. According to Sciencedaily.com, there are a lot of researches proving the pet parents have lower blood pressure, less anxiety, and experience lifts in their depression. One study actually proved that with a little than 10 minutes, a pet can lower blood pressure significantly.

Pet parents even have overall better physical health due to exercise with their pets. Actually senior, citizens who own pets actually need less medical attention. Not only are sick and old people benefits from pets. Children exposed to pets during their first year of life have a lower frequency of asthma and allergies.

Pet parents who have undergone surgery even have lower recovery time. There is even a study saying that heart attack patients with pets have longer life expectancy than those who do not. There is even a study saying that pets decrease heart attack mortality rates by 3 percent which is 30,0000 lives every year. HIV/AIDS victims who have pets also report less depression and can reduce stress levels.

There are countless research proving that taking an animal into their homes is a great way to enhance their personal and family health. The love and care that pet parents provide to their pets in indeed reciprocated. Aside from humane and health benefits that pet adoption can give, it is also a great way of saving money.

For a price which is very much less compared to pet store pets, you will get an animal that will be able to provide you with loyalty and devotion.

Pet Adoption Considerations - Are You Fit to be a Pet Owner?

In any decision that you do in life, you must think hard about it in order to arrive at the best choice as much as possible. In the end, it is also you who will suffer or who will benefit from anything that will arise from that. Pet adoption considerations must also be at the top of your mind if you want to venture into this situation.

Why would you want to adopt?

Your reasons can be as simple as you want to gain a companion. The pets of your choice will depend on your lifestyle. You don't want to get an animal that will require a lot from you physically if you cannot really afford the time to give it to them. You can just settle for a tamer one like a fish, rabbit or parrot that will serve as a companion white they really don't ask you for too much attention. It will be enough for you to give them their basic necessities like shelter, warmth and food.

You may also want to acquire a pet because you merely want to make a difference and help in this good cause. You may have a soft spot for animals especially for those that have been left in shelters or have been cared for by charitable institutions. This is a good omen and can lead you towards a brighter future in caring for pets. Just make sure that you are ready for the responsibilities that will be required from you when you opt to trek this route.

Do not give pets as presents.

This is a must. The reason for this is very obvious. The recipient of the gift may not be ready to owe up to the responsibilities that your gift comes with. What do you think will happen to the animal when they are handed to an unwilling owner? You may have your own reasons why you give the pets as gifts. You may think that you've already assessed the recipient based on the facts that you know about them. But for sure, there are certain spots that you do not know about them. The pets may end up in shelters or may also be given out to others. The worst thing that could happen is for the pet to be ignored and may cause its health to diminish.

What are the other considerations?

Owning pets will give you lots of joy. But these are animals. You cannot teach them to tidy up by themselves. So expect the unexpected. Prepare yourself to clean up your pet's mess that may be distributed even on your favorite parts of your house. You can teach your pets tricks and share with them some manners. But you must not expect them to follow what you are saying all the time. They may be intelligent but you are superior than they are. You cannot expect them to do the right things all the time. You may be surprised to see eaten foods or chewed papers or shoes at times.

If you are not prepared for such situation, what are you going to do? The most probable thing is that you will vent your anger at your pet. You may want to decide to get lost of them the instant they did what seems to be inexplicable. These pet adoption considerations can help you open your eyes and mind if you can be trusted to be a responsible pet owner.

Pet Adoption Fees

Pet adoption fees are being collected during the adoption fees. Whether it is a pet adoption from shelters or from rescue groups, adoption fees range from $75 dollars to $200 dollars. There have been numerous debates over pet adoption fees.

People who are giving up their pet for adoption think that their pets are not up for adoption but for sale. Most people think that it is inappropriate to charge for an animal that is already homeless or soon to be homeless. Some people interpret that shelters and rescue groups are in it for the money, rather than looking for the best suitable home for their beloved pets.

There are even arguments from people saying that the range of the adoption fee is too high, something between $20 to $50 dollars will be suitable enough for "homeless" animals. The higher the adoption fee, the larger is the misconception that organizations and people are just trying to get money from other people's pockets.

But there are realistic reasons for charging an adoption fee. Adoption fees make sure that animals are going to suitable, responsible and secure homes.

It is a sad reality that there are dog fighting rings and animals can be used as bait to train fighting dogs. Giving away animals can make these "homeless" animals more vulnerable to abuse.

Paying adoption fees also shows commitment. If there are people who are unable to pay for their pet's adoption fees, how likely is it that these people will provide for their pet's other needs. Pets do not only require attention and time, but also they require financial responsibility. Aside from food, grooming and day-to-day needs, there are also regular veterinary check-ups and vaccines that needs to be done.

Pet adoption fees do not go to people's pockets for personal use. Pet adoption fees cover the operating expenses, pet care, medical bills and so forth. In most cases, adoption fees may also fall short of the actual expenses.

Pet adoption fee is sometimes determined by the vetting cost. This include vaccinations (for puppies normally it takes over a period of 6 weeks to 16 weeks) and spay/neuter. There are even adoptable animals that require dental cleaning or tooth removal or a surgery. Still, shelters and rescue groups do not overcharge and still go with the normal fee.

For animal rescue groups, their adoption fees are usually higher than that of shelters. Shelters often have relationship with rescue groups, they ask rescue groups to take responsibility for animals that they cannot afford to pay for the vetting cost.

There are people who are doing the adoption process personally without shelter or animal rescue organization help to ensure that their pets will be taken to a good home. Individual pet owners may charge adoption fee since there are times that they include kennel, food dishes, toys, bedding and other pet accessories before adopting. Some would require an adoption fee to cover the vetting costs that they have incurred while taking responsibility for the pet.

Why animal rescue groups charge higher fees than shelters is that are volunteers that provide care and training for animals using their own personal finances. Rescue groups do not have corporate backing. Rescuers use their funds for looking up on the best possible match, setting up conveyance when needed, calling adopting family prospects and reference checks.

Pet adoption fees are justified by having a healthy companion or additional family member. Let's remember that pets are not toys to be discarded when we are already done with playing them.

The sad truth is since we are living in a material world, pets without value are considered disposable.

Pet Adoption from Rescue Groups

Rescue groups or organizations are volunteer groups dedicated to pet adoption. These groups or organizations take the unwanted, abandoned, abused and stray animals and attempt to locate life long homes for these animals. Rescue groups may also take the animals themselves and care for them, providing them training, medical care and taking care of the behavioural problems until they get a suitable home for them.

Pet adoption from rescue groups is a great way of providing a loving home for pets that may not have any owners or any loving and caring experience. Rescue animals just need a little bit more of guidance and stable environment.

Rescue animals, most of the time, have spent time in a family environment. So some of the rescue animals have already gone some obedience training and already housebroken. Although there is still some rescue animals, due to owner's neglect haven't gone any training at all. Rescue groups make sure that animals have been housebroken or trained before being put up for adoption.

Also, rescue organizations are including temperament testing in their processes before accepting a pet into their programs. Foster families or soon-to-be-parents of the rescued animals have the opportunity to continue in observing the behaviour of animals before being available for adoption. With this process, the soon-to-be-pet parents can make an informed decision if they will be able to cope with the behaviour and attitude of the rescue animals.

In terms of medical care, rescue animals if already old enough, may have already been neutered and received vaccinations. Rescue pets have already undergone physical examination. If there are some health issues, they have been treated while in foster care. Health problems are being taken care of prior to adoption.

The bond between rescue animals and their pet owners are very strong. It is commonly noticed and shared that rescue animals are eager to please their new owners. They are usually eager to be part of a loving family where they know they are safe and secure.

Animals that have experienced abuse and neglect when shown or treated with kindness become devoted, loving and loyal companions. Skittish and timid animals become more confident eventually becoming more affectionate and outgoing. There are experiences from rescued puppies to wanting to be in their new owner's lap and following them at all times.

Rescue organizations are very keen of placing their animals in suitable homes that will be their life long or "forever" home. Pet parents looking to adopt for pets undergo a selection process that will make sure that the pet is suitable to the type of family doing the adoption. If ever the family encounters a problem that cannot be given a solution, most rescue groups have a return clause written in their adoption contract.

But generally, adult pets that you can get from the rescue groups are better adapting to their new family especially kids. Housebroken and adult pets are more mellow and more patient with children.

Adopting a pet is a good value that can be though to our children. Especially since everything can be bought, adopting provides a great opportunity to teach our children compassion, caring , second chances and responsibility.

If pet parents are interested getting purebred dogs, there are purebred rescue groups. These rescue groups are voluntarily run by people with in-depth knowledge of a specific breed. Adopting fees vary depending on the veterinary and medical costs that have been spent while they are in foster care. Follow-up counselling is also available for post adoption problems.

Rescue groups and organizations provide the opportunity for animals to be relocated in much secure and safe homes. Pet adoption is a great and humane thing to do.

Shelter Pets: Pet Adoption Myths

Pet adoption is a great way of getting pets in a much less price. Pet adoption is also a great way of taking care and proving homes for pets and animals that have been left or sometimes even abused by their previous owners.

Adopting pets from shelters just charge an adoption fee which is very far from the regular prices of animals in pet stores. Adoption fees range from $35 to $200 and almost always include medical treatment like vaccines, deworming, and spaying (neuter). There are even shelters that offer follow up veterinary services to ensure that pets remain healthy and able to get the necessary vaccines.

Animal shelters provide great choices for adoptable pets. Shelters not only have adult animals, but they also have kittens and puppies that a pet parent can choose from. However there are some myths about animal shelters and why it is not a good place to adopt from.

Many people believe that pets in shelters have behavioural problems. It is important to remember that these animals have bad experiences from their previous owners. They might have experienced neglect and abuse. Animals in shelters normally exhibit minor behavioural problems. Some of these pets may be scared while others can be excited. Animals that show major behavioural problems are not put up for adoption.

Animal shelters perform screen test to know the temperament of animals in the shelters. The shelters try to get as much information they could get from the animals' previous owners. Soon-to-be pet parents are happier and at ease to know that their new pet has healthy and friendly temperament.

Since these animals have been neglected, abused and abandoned, the next parent should display more patience to train them. Also since these pets already know and encountered difficult hardships they display more loyalty and devotion to their new owners. There are some pet parents who have adopted from shelters saying that their pets are more loyal and loving than other pets.

Another shelter myth says that pets from shelters and pounds are mature animals and cannot be trained. Most pets in shelter are older animals but there are also kittens and puppies that is available for adoption.

Adoptable animals from shelters can be trained like other animals. The important thing during training is to be consistent, patient and understanding. Animals (regardless if they are in shelter or in homes) respond to good, effective, loving and humane training techniques.

There are shelters that offer the new pet parent the opportunity to participate in obedience training and pet parenting classes. These sessions serve as a transition period for the pet and the parent to bond together.

It is commonly believed that pets in animal shelters are inferior to purebred animals. According to the Humane Society of the United States there is an average of 25 to 30 per cent of purebreds in animal shelters.

Also, mixed bred animals are not inferior to purebred animals. Animal shelters have pets that are healthier and have better temperaments than purebred. Interested pet parents just have to talk to the shelter and provide the what kind of behaviour they would like to have in their pets. Mixed bred pets oftentimes exhibit traits of several breeds. If a pet parent like to have a purebred because of its temperament, the shelter would likely have a mixed bred that exhibits the qualities of the purebred.

Going to a shelter for a pet adoption is a great way of helping animals in need in a much affordable and economic way. Adopting a pet from a shelter is not only a solution for the pet parent's problem but also a way of saving a life.

The Pet Adoption Process

There are many myths about the pet adoption. Several myths about pet adoption is that the parent or adult will get an animal with behavioural problems or temperament which may not suit the family. There is also an animal shelter myth saying that animals in shelters are less valuable or intelligent that purebred animals.

To eradicate our fears of these pet adoption myths, we should know the adoption and selection process done by animal rescue groups and shelters. We should be wholly participative in the adoption process to make a success out of the pet adoption.

Rescue groups and shelters ask a lot of questions about the prospective pet parents or adopters. There are two reasons for this: first, is to be sure that the adopter will be able to provide the new pet a permanent home and if the adopter is capable of the responsibility and financial commitment a pet requires. The other reason is to ensure that the adopter and the pet would have a good match. They normally do it interviews or signing application forms.

The best way to be sure what kind of pet the adopter is interested in having, is by carrying out research of their own. There are several questions that will help the adopter to determine the pet, like activeness, family composition, type of residence, or love for the outdoors.

There are several websites that displays different animal characteristics and one the choice had been made, the adopter can inform the shelter or rescuers what animal they have in mind. Shelter and rescuers can identify what breed of animals you might be interested in. Also they have a selection of mixed bred pets that can also display the characteristics of an animal or pet you have in mind.

Some of the questions may even be intrusive of the adopter's personal life, but the rescuers and shelter staff are just trying to make sure that these homeless animals' interest will be top priority. Another step that can be done to assist the adopter to be prepared with what to expect in the adoption process is by checking the websites of shelters and rescue groups.

There are also some shelters and rescuers that do a "yard check" before the pets are taken to their new homes. It is quite necessary since shelters and rescue groups have full grown animals that need a larger size of place to roam and have physical activities.

Some even do veterinary check with the present or former vet clinics. This is to ensure that current of previous pets were up-to-date with their shots, exams and other medical attention they require. While there are others who require three character references in their application papers, aside from the veterinary to be really sure.

After these have been completed with both parties satisfied, an adoption contract is presented as a final step in the process. An adoption contract contains information such as required veterinary visits, vaccination, a required spay/neuter, diet, continuation of medical treatments of prescription (if necessary) and return clauses if the owner no longer wishes to take care of the animal.

To fully adopt the animal, a pet adoption fee is needed to conclude the process. Normally the price ranges from $75 to $200 dollars depending on the size, animal, and vetting costs. After this, adopters and now-pet-parents get to take home their beloved pets.

Pet Adoption: Things to Consider Before Adopting

Everybody, sometime in a point of their lives, were taken by pets who are looking at us with cute eyes begging for attention or a little pat on the head. They may be in a pet shop that we just passed by or in a shelter. No matter where we found them, once we see "the look", the next thing we know, this pet is already messing your bedroom floor.

Having a pet at home is a wonderful experience, whether it is for the whole family or for an individual. However, having a pet, more so, adopting a pet to live with us is a big decision. It is important to know first our capabilities in caring for a pet.

The Humane Society of the United States formulated some questions to answer before pursuing any plans of pet adoption. According to them, we would have to consider the reason for adopting. It is important to know why we are adopting, failing to answer or provide a good answer for this could lead to a big mistake.

Pets and animal companions just cannot be ignored. It is important to know if we would have time to spend caring a pet. Pets put up for adoptions are mostly in shelters. Let us remember that these pets were put into shelters because their owners can no longer take care of them.

Pet or animal care is very expensive nowadays. Pets not only require water and food but also they need to undergo training, grooming and other expenses. Let us remember that these pets are not only staying overnight or for a week. Pets can live with us from 10 until 20 years. It is important to know if we can afford to let a pet into our lives. We need to know and answer if we can be responsible pet owners.

Pets of course, bring good things like joy and love in the house. But aside from these, pets are also bearers of infestations, damaged furniture, accidents from animals not yet trained and unexpected medical emergencies. Knowing our ability to cope and resolve this issue are important concerns to be addressed to. Meanwhile, if ever you choose to go to a vacation, it is necessary to look for somebody to take charge of the pets while away.

Research is good thing. It is necessary to research about the animals that we are interested in adopting. We need to know about their characteristics to arrange their stay.

It is absolutely necessary to know if any members of the family or companions in the house have allergy towards certain breed of pets. If ever there are children in the family, with ages below six, it is important to rethink the adoption. Pets require responsibility so it may be difficult for the children to take responsibility of the pet. It is better to let a few years go by before getting another animal.

If there is another pet at home, it is important to consider if the new pet will get along with the other animal. Having a veterinarian is also important in caring for out pet animals.

There are certain places that have rules about the leash use on animals. There are also places that have local provisions about the most number of pets a person can own. Sometimes they even require the owner to have pet licenses.

Whether it is pet adoption or just simple pet ownership, it requires a lot of patience and care for our animals. It is important to answer the mention considerations before proceeding in getting pets.

Pet Adoption Tips – Helping You Arrive with the Right Decision

Are you the kind of person who wants to give back to the goodness that life is bringing your way? Or are you just compassionate and care about any living thing? Maybe you were born or raised as a pet lover. If you want pet adoption tips that can help you in deciding whether this is the right time to do this or not, the first thing that you have to remember is to listen closely to your heart.

Is this really what you want to happen? Why do you want this? If you already own a pet, why would you still want to adopt an additional? You may think that there are too many questions being posed with the simple query about tips. But these questions are vital if you want to succeed in this venture.

Imagine this. There are many uncared for animals roaming aimlessly at this cruel world. You may have seen the news about other nations, states and localities doing unimaginable things to these animals. But in the first place, why did these pets end up in the streets with no food, no shelter and no one to take care of them?

Lost Pets
One reason could be the undecided people who thought that they can handle the responsibilities of being a pet owner after they have gone through the adoption process. It is really hard in all aspects. Pet ownership requires a lot from you. Physically, you have to provide fun and enjoyment to your pets by having them participate on activities. Or you can merely play with them or walk them around the neighbourhood at night or job with them during the day. Emotionally, you have to really care about the animals to ensure that you have only their well-being in mind. You've got to attach to them on this level so that your pet will feel wanted and loved. And financially, you have to allot a budget for instances wherein your pets may suffer from certain illnesses or may be in some sort of accidents.

Another reason for pets to appear lost is that they may really have gotten lost. This scenario cannot be helped. It will be good if you can find their rightful owner. The latter will surely be grateful, especially if they think of their pets as part of their family. But it will be hard to do so when you don't have the means. As much as you want to help the pet to come back to its rightful owner, you can place it on a shelter that can provide them the necessities or you can agree on the responsibility of owning it and treating the pet as a family.

And when pet owners die, who do you think will care for their pets? If the other relatives of family members will not owe up to the responsibility, the pet may choose to wander while wondering where their owners go. Or maybe they are also in search for new owners to find them and care for them like how their former companion treated them.

Make a Move
In order for you to decide whether you will adopt or not, here are some tips that you may want to look into.

1. Make sure that you talk about your plan to your family and everybody who is living in the house with you. They deserve to know about it beforehand so they can give their suggestions regarding the matter.

2. You have to be prepared to be a responsible pet owner.

3. And the last of these pet adoption tips is to find the right link that will point you to the right pet that will suit your preference and will fit perfectly into your life.

Reasons for Pet Adoption - Are You Ready to Become a Pet Owner?

The reasons for pet adoption can be as varied as your choices during the springtime and early fall in centres and shelters. These are known as the breeding season. And because of that fact, people who will choose to adopt during this period will have lots of animals to choose from, different types, different kinds, breeds, sizes. You name it. You will have a breeze in finding the right pet that will be a welcome sight to your home and to your life.

Pet adoption can be achieved through lots of ways. The setup can be a formal one, like you will go to a shelter and sign the necessary papers for your chosen pet to be released. You will go through all the necessary process from choosing the pets to assisting on legal documents that other localities may want you to accomplish. Other centers will ask you for a minimal fee. In return, you are assured that the animal that you will be getting is free of any sickness and have been treated with the right medication and proper vaccinations.

You can also find online pet adoption portals that can give you choices of animals that you can adopt for free. These are usually owned by charitable institutions that aim to help the needy animals to find shelter and families for them. At this instance, you have to take the initiative to bring the animal that you have chosen to your local vet to be treated or vaccinated. You have to ensure that the pet is healthy before you bring it home.

The charitable institutions have only the best intentions for these animals. But you cannot blame them if they cannot afford to bring the animals to the vets as required. They work hard to find sponsors. But with the numbers of pets being sent to them each day, they need your help to accomplish the rest of the procedure to make sure that the animal will live long.

You can also adopt informally. Like for example, you know a pet owner who will be moving out of the country for justifiable reasons. Or you know someone who can no longer afford the responsibilities of taking care of their pets because of lack of finances. You can talk it out with them. You can adopt their pets for free. Or if they opt to sell it, you can also think hard about it. In any case, you have to look closely at the pet. Is this the type that you will be able to handle? Or are just going to cost more sufferings to the animal? If the latter is the case, then it will be better if you will advice the owners to send the animals to shelters or to charitable institutions or even to local vets who may have links with these associations.

The Reasons
So what motivates you to own a pet? Look at this list and determine if you are ready for the challenges that it may pose. This will also help you decide what kind of pets will be beneficial to the kind of setup that you have at home and at your overall lifestyle.

1. You want a companion from a stressful and busy life. If you don't have much time to spare, you may

want to opt for animals that will not require so much from you. You may want to look into rabbits. You may also want a bird that is easy to maintain. You also can contemplate about owning a fish. Remember that your pets must suit your lifestyle.

2. You want to help. This is a good cause that you can participate to. But if you don't really have the time to spare to be a responsible pet owner, you can just donate goods or cash to the charities or shelters that care for these animals.

So what are your reasons for pet adoption? Hear yourself out. If you can convince your heart that this is the right thing to do, then maybe this really is for you.

Saving Our Furry Friends through Pet Adoptions

Did you know that in pet adoptions centers, animals have an expiration date? The staff of animal shelters put animals to sleep after a specified duration of time, if they don't get adopted. We really can't blame the shelters for this; it is a legal though upsetting procedure they have to carry out.

There are a few reasons why animals must be put to sleep when no one adopts them:

* One of the most common problems in animal shelters is the lack of space. Stray or abandoned animals are sheltered for a specific number of days before they can be put into adoption program or, sadly, put to sleep. This gives the owner of the animals ample time to find and reclaim their furry friends. Remember that during the holding period of an animal, newer ones are continually being brought to the animal shelter.

* Not all of the animals brought to animal shelters are in good health and adoptable condition. Sometimes an animal is brought in that's unwell and mentally unstable. Should the animal shelter's staff deem the animal cannot be helped or adopted, it is put to sleep right away.

* In some cases, an animal that has been in the animal shelter for too long may exhibit signs of stress. Behaviours such as agitation, anxiety, depression and aggression begin to show up, which is not typical for the animal. In the long run, if the animal does not get adopted, it becomes so mentally

unsound that the staff of the animal shelter has to put it to sleep.

The pros of adopting from shelters

The best way to prevent these animals in shelters from being put to sleep is by adopting them. Whether you are planning to own a dog, cat, ferrets or any other animal, you are not only saving their lives but you are also getting a loyal companion for yourself.

What makes adopting an animal from an animal shelter is that you know what you will be taking home with you. Our furry friends in animal shelters have been examined by veterinarians. This means that the animal you'll be getting is up to date with its shots, and its medical condition is properly looked over. Animal shelters may sometimes charge a fee for adoption, but still it's a lot cheaper than buying a new one from pet stores, or compared to the service they had provided for the animal.

Taking your time in picking one

Be sure to take your time looking around and choose the healthiest animal you can find in an animal shelter. Look for one with ears and nose that are clean and free of mucous. The eyes should be bright and clear. Carefully inspect its coat and skin; look carefully for signs sores, bald spots or skin diseases. Also check the way they walk – they should not be limping, which gives away skeletal problems such as deformities and fractures.

Adopting an animal from pet adoptions centers means you are willing to bestow time and dedication in taking care of a furry friend. Remember that you will have other expenses besides the adoption charge itself. But all these are a small price to pay for saving the life of an animal and earning a loyal companion for the rest of its natural life.

Pet Adoption Verdict: Adopting the Best Companion for You

Pet adoption should never be done spontaneously. There are numerous reasons why pets are being surrendered in shelters and rescue organization, most common reason is deciding spontaneously about getting a pet and then failing to do the responsibility that taking care of pets requires.

Therefore, before adopting an animal from rescuers or shelters it is important that the animal that you are choosing will be a life-long companion. Otherwise, this defeats the mission and goal of animal shelters and animal rescue organizations.

Shelters and rescue groups have wide selection of puppies and full-grown cats and dogs. It is important to identify which animal will be most suitable for the adopter's personality and temperament. Adoptable cats and dogs (whether purebred or mixed bred) displays different characteristics. It is best not to rely only on the physical characteristics of these animals but focus more on their attitude and behaviour.

Choosing Your Feline Companion

Cats make wonderful pets. Although they value their independence, they crave for love and companionship. What is good about cats is that they can easily adjust to different lifestyles and types of residences.

When choosing cats in an animal shelter, it is best to ask permission or assistance from the adoption counsellor to spend some time with the animals. This is to better understand the behaviour and temperament of the animals. Although, keep in mind that since it is an unfamiliar environment for the animals, there are cats that tend to be timid, passive or frightened even if they are naturally sociable.

Having young children at home is another thing to consider. Young children usually cannot handle the responsibility of kittens. A cat, at least four months old will be a good choice.

If the adopter have other animals at home, it is best to help the new member of the family to adjust to its surroundings. Adopters can try isolating their new cats in a room and then slowly exposing them to the other animals. With this, they can slowly associate with each other until they accept the new cat's presence in the house.

Choosing the Best Dog

Adopters sometimes get overwhelmed with the wide selection of purebreds and mixed bred animals in shelters. The best way to narrow down the choices is identifying the adopter's characteristics or personality. Another thing is learning about the different personalities and temperaments of purebreds and mixes.

With this process, you can do a process of elimination by removing those breeds and mixes that do not match or complement the adopter's lifestyle.

When visiting animals in shelters; always keep in mind that this is a stressful and unfamiliar environment for the dogs. The dog's true character will be best displayed if they are in a secure and safe place.

Again, ask for the adoption counsellor's attention to known several information about the dogs you are interested. Ask the age, the behaviour, and if the animal is good with children. It is important to narrow down the choices before going to shelter, this also applies for cat adoption.

Remember that the pets that you are adopting will be your companion for the next 10 until 15 years – or even longer. That's why it is important for adopter's to carefully choose their ideal pet. Pet adoption makes the most wonderful unions between pets and owners, as long as the decisions were made in no rush and with guidance.

Pet Adoption Versus Animal Euthanasia

Animal euthanasia is the act of inducing death to an animal. Euthanasia methods are designed to cause minimal pain and distress. Most of the times, it is called the act of "putting asleep" an animal. Meanwhile organizations like animal rescue groups and animal rights organizations strictly oppose this method. They say pet adoption could dramatically reduce the number of animals being "put to sleep".

There are many reasons for animal euthanasia. Terminal illness, behavioural problems like aggression can be reasons for euthanasia. While there are animal owners inducing their animals or pets to euthanasia when they have illnesses or broken limbs that require medical attention and require financial aid.

Old age is also a common reason for animal or pet euthanasia. Meanwhile for animal shelters, they induce euthanasia since they do not have enough space or room for an abandoned animal.

According to Humane Society of the United States, there is an estimated 4 to 5 million of adoptable animals in animal shelters euthanized due to lack of facilities. While American Humane Association cites even a bigger number, 9.6 million of animals in the United States are being euthanized every year.

According to the survey conducted by the American Humane Association, out of the 1000 shelters who responded to the survey, 2.7 million of 4.3 million animals (64 per cent) are being euthanized. Out of this euthanized number, 56 per cent are dogs and 71 per cent are cats. There 15 per cent of dogs and 2 per cent of cars were reunited with their owners. Just a dismal 25 per cent of dogs and 24 per cent of cats were adopted.

Majority of the animals in shelters were being euthanized since there is a standard period of time (ranging from several days to weeks for unclaimed stray animals). However, there are "no kill" shelters run by private and animal welfare organizations. These "no kill" shelters make it an official policy never to euthanize animals for medical reasons.

Another reason why animal euthanasia is creeping to our culture is because of pet overpopulation. There are numerous pet owners surrendering their pet due to personal reasons and inadequacy in taking responsibility for their pets. There are also people who only wants puppies, once the puppies grow, they completely neglect them and eventually surrender them to shelters or rescue groups.

There are owners who due to failure of spaying or neutering their animals tend to reproduce. There are thousands of litters being born in American homes every day. It is important to consider the financial and medical attention and responsibility these huge numbers of pet reproduction. We do not want to contribute to the raising number of people surrendering their pets for adoption. Eventually, this will lead to pets not being adopted and eventually pet euthanasia.

Clearly, there is crisis in the pet population of the United States. Too many animal companions competing for a few good homes than will take them is a clear effect of uncontrolled breeding.

Dog bite victims are now ranging to 4.5 million each year, due to uncontrolled breeding. Some of the victims fall prey to homeless and stray animals in the streets. They pose public danger, and the government is paying the people's tax money in controlling these animals and maintaining animal shelters.

Pet adoption is a great way of lessening the impact of the crisis in pet population. Instead of buying pets from puppy mills or companies that breeds animals for profit, adopting an animal is a great way of reducing the number of euthanized animals in shelters.

There are countless benefits of pet adoption. There are studies conducted saying the adopted pets are more loyal and devoted since they have already experienced the worst. Pet adoption is a great way of reducing the number of animals in shelters and making way for another one. Pet adoption battles euthanasia – one pet at a time.

Significant Facts about Pet Adoptions

Have you ever thought about going through the available options for pet adoptions? Pet lovers need not worry about finding the right furry companion for them. They are available everywhere, even on the cyberspace. But you must remember that owning pets entails lots of responsibilities. Here are some notes that can guide you before you decide on becoming a full-fledged pet owner.

1. Adopting is less expensive than buying a pet. The cost will depend on the type of adoption center where you will be getting the pets. There are some places, just to give you a sample of how much it would cost, you could get a puppy for $150. If you opt to buy this, the prices usually range from $300 up to $600. Your expenses don't stop there. You have to pay for the puppy's vaccinations for its first years which may be about $150 up to $300. Other health tests must also be accomplished to ensure your pet's health. This will cost you about $50 up to $200.

2. You are confident that you are getting a healthy animal as a pet. When you opt to adopt a puppy, the case is usually like this. The animal shelter will assure you that it already has gone through thorough examinations. And what are these? First, your puppy's fleas have already been treated. You just have to maintain that in order to keep your companion well groomed. Health examinations for the puppy have already been done by the center and they make sure that before you get the animal, it has passed all tests. This assures you that you are getting a healthy pup.

If it is already suitable, when the animal is on its right age, the center will also provide its needed vaccinations. They also test the pups for parvovirus and some also do some testing for heart worm. Heart worm, distemper and parvo-influenza are considered terminal diseases for dogs. So you have to make sure that your pet have gone through tests for these and passed them all.

And this situation applies to all animals in your chosen shelter. They are all being given attention and proper funding to look out for their health.

3. When you are on the process of adopting a pet, you will be assisted by the center's staff so that they can match you with the right animal. And this process is also extremely important. This is like helping you find the perfect partner or the additional family member who would be accepted by the family. If you'd like to get a dog, there are many kinds of dogs not only in terms of breed but also with the attitude.

You will find purebred and cross-bred dogs of different sizes and personalities. There are those that are shy and others with extremely high energy. You will be asked by the center if you are the type of person who loves sports and may want to bring the pet on your running sessions. Or are you the type who just wants to stay home after a stressful day and be comforted by the fact that you are no longer alone.

Pet adoptions can be fun as well as challenging. But you have to be responsible for the pet's well-being after you have left the shelter. So make sure that you have thought about it real hard and you are ready to commit to the idea that you will be answerable to whatever will happen to your chosen pet once you have taken it home.

Some Vital Cautions on Pet Adoption

Are you the type of person who loves giving surprises? Are you the kind who will try hard to think how are you going to make your loved ones feel that they are special? If you are pulling the trick all the time, you may feel that you are already running out of ideas. There is one surprise that you must not opt for. And this is none other than pet adoption.

Advantages of Pet Ownership
There are a lot of advantages of owning pets. It doesn't matter whether you are still young or you are on your senior years. Pets bring lots of joys in people's lives. But the kind of pet that one must own should be according to their lifestyle. So how can pets change people's lives? Here are only some of the reasons.

1. Companionship is the first and most popular reason whether for old and young people. They get pets of their choice to be there as a friend or even as a family. You treat your pets like babies. You feed them, bathe them and even teach them tricks if you can. For over stressed individuals and those who do not have their families to greet them upon coming home, pets become their alternative for such purpose.

2. There are scientific studies which proved that pets can cause good effects on one's heath, especially with the elders. Owning one and interacting with them can reduce your cholesterol levels. It can also regulate your blood pressure. Of

course, it can eliminate or reduce the stress levels that you are feeling. Others say that this can also prevent some cardiovascular diseases from recurring.

Overall, owning pets can lead to a healthier you. Plus, you will also be happier and more energized. You will get the sense of responsibility for your pets' health and lives. You will have fun, excitement and more alert.

Red Alert

But not because you've read about the advantages of owning a pet means that you will head out the nearest adoption center and surprise someone with one. Mind you, this will also come with a lot of responsibility which the recipient may not be ready to owe up to. So make sure that you talk first to the person you have in mind to give a pet to before you make any moves.

1. Do not give those who are not asking for it. There are reasons why people choose to have pets. But there are also reasons why they opt not to. This is the basis why the American Humane Society advices people to discuss the matter with the would-be owner before you pass on to them the responsibility of owning a pet. They do not encourage the gesture of giving pets as gifts.

2. Discussing will also prove to be easier on both parties. If they really want to own pets, at least you can ask them for their preferences. This way, you are assured that when you give them the pets, they will be happy about the gesture and that they will be prepared to care for the animal.

The vital factor in pet adoption is that you have to find the perfect match between owners and the pets. You have to make sure that both will like and love the fate that they are both about to venture into.

Virtual Pet Adoption – Teaching Kids about Responsibility

Having a loving pet in the family can be a real joy. Pets make good companions and they can become real members of the family. If your kids have never experienced having a pet before, but would like to have one, you may find that virtual pet adoption can give them that know-how. It can help let your little ones experience what it is like to have a real pet of their own.

Unfortunately, kids often yearn for having a pet with little or no idea of what it really takes to take care of one. The responsibility of having an animal in the house is not as easy as it may sound like. Often the attention it demands can interfere with day to day living and can be too demanding. But once a bond has been formed with a pet, it becomes awfully difficult not to take care of it properly; you have no choice but to get on with the responsibilities of owning one as best as you can.

A whole lot like real pets

What makes owning a computer generated pet such a good idea for your kids? Well, as your little ones are taking care of their adopted virtual pet, they learn about what it would be like to take care of a real animal. Just like a real pet, your children will also have to perform a few things to their virtual ones as they take care of them. These artificial companions are replicas of real animals, so they basically seek the same kind of interaction from their owners as real pets.

Getting your kids to pick and look after their virtual furry companion will give them the same satisfaction they get from owning a real pet. They will get to name their chosen pets, feed them when they become hungry, ensure that they have enough water to drink, buy them stuff, play with them, and even take them out. Plus your little ones will also get the positive feedback from their simulated pets if they're satisfied with how they're taken care of – just like a real pet.

Picking the best one for the family

Does your child want a golden retriever, a Persian cat, a cockatoo or a python perhaps? There are a great variety of virtual pets your kids may adopt. Some of the available animals children can pet on their computer include cats, dogs, birds, mice, turtles, snakes, monkeys, fishes and many more. But they can also opt for a few unconventional creatures to take care of, like monsters or aliens.

The good thing about getting your kids to adopt a virtual pet before buying an actual one for the family is to test if it's the animal suited for your household. For instance, if you think that a cat is the perfect companion around the house, you can try looking after one in a simulated manner first.

Taking care of a pet is like taking care of a true member of the family. It requires time, love and devotion; and a lot of patience and practice to. The best way to instill and develop a sense of responsibility in your little ones in taking care of pets is to trough virtual pet adoption. Your kids will have a great time looking after them as they get ready to get a real pet of their own.

LINKS FOR PET ADOPTION

Far Place
http://www.farplace.org.uk/

Animal Rescue and Care
http://www.animalrescueandcare.org.uk/

Battersea Dogs and Cats
http://www.battersea.org.uk/

RSPCA
http://www.rspca.org.uk/home

Pets at Home
http://www.petsathome.com/

Pet Finder
http://www.petfinder.com/index.html

Adopt a Pet
http://www.adoptapet.com/

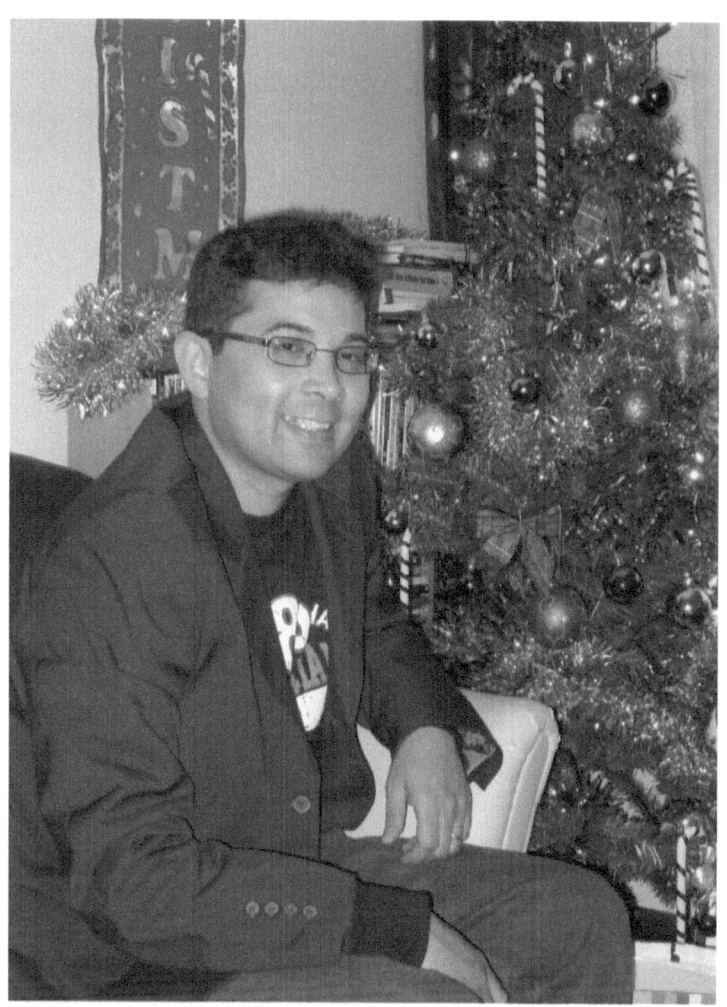

ABOUT THE AUTHOR

Warren Brown is an Amazon published Author, freelance writer, journalist, copywriter, proof-reader, Law of Attraction Practitioner and Life Coach.

http://www.publishsuccess.com

http://warrenbrown.blogspot.com

Email: info@publishsuccess.com

Researched, compiled and Edited by Warren Brown.

Copyright @Warren Brown

ISBN 978-1-291-22708-6

London. United Kingdom.2012